On the **Sunny Side** of the Street.

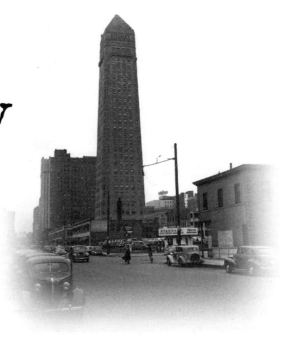

An Alzheimer's Journey

Christine Fournier

Beaver's Pond Press, Inc.

ISBN 1-931646-16-3

Library of Congress Catalog Number: 2001096150

Printed in the United States of America.

05 04 03 02 01   6 5 4 3 2 1

Beaver's Pond Press, Inc.

5125 Danen's Drive
Edina, MN 55439-1465
(952) 829-8818
www.beaverspondpress.com

On October 23, 1996, my mother Helen Winter LaCaze passed away due to complications from Alzheimer's Disease. This memoir is dedicated to her, the estimated twenty-two million people who will be afflicted by this devastating disease in this century, and to the family caregivers and professional health care workers who will usher them through this journey.

Christine Fournier
December, 2001

For Dale:
Best wishes and love to you on your journey.
Christine Fournier

Table
of
Contents

Acknowledgments

T he following people and organizations gave advice, support, time, and unconditional love during a difficult and challenging period of years. To all of you I extend my gratitude and love.

The Alzheimer's Association, Minnesota-Dakotas Chapter; St. Louis Park Plaza Care Facility; Walker Place Care Facility; Park-Nicollet Senior Services; Altercare; Metro Mobility of the Twin Cities; Ebenezer Luther Hall; The Cremation Society of Minnesota; Siddha Yoga Meditation Center of The Twin Cities; Nemer, Fieger and Associates, Inc.; Al-Anon 54th Street Family Group; Order of Eastern Star, Lake Harriet Chapter of the Twin Cities; Zuhrah Shrine Temple Ladie's Auxiliary; Mike Lorenz; Kristi Vrieze; Vera West; Fran Eng; Kelly Leonard; Gloria Pinsky; Donna Ware; Leslie Hart; Sharon Sewall; Phyllis Gamble; Jeanne Johnson; Betty Roman and Gretchen Benda; Janet Foster; Ellie Bisek; Dr. Sharon Marx; Cheryl Biel; Bobbi Speich; Julie Nygren; Barbara Holmquist; Kordie Reinhold, D.D.S.; Rhonda Altom, DOS; Joyce Fowler; Martha Schaefer; Marion and Carr Hagerman; Aaron and Nancy Houseman; Judge Herbert Lefler; Attorney Mark Douglass; Chris Conangla; KSTP Television; the entire Winter family; Jim and June Fieger; The Meline family; Kitty Larson; Jerry Stamm; Greg Fandel; Mike and Barbara Walter; Betsy and Tom Dodder; Christopher Ruhl and Susan Lucey; Barbara Cogelow; Isabel Goepferd; Mike Freeman; Rachel Henke; Michael Tracy; David Bryce; Jackie Steele; Jimmy Martin; John Command; Daniel Crawford; Mardi Grant; J.B. Davidson; Joel Thom; Toni and Bill

Souza; Brooke Roma; Ron and Courtney Roberts; Dr. Debbra Ford; Pastor David Englestad; Janet Crownover; Barbara and Tom Hurley; Eric Vevea; Rex Thompson; Eric Loeffler; and Joan and Phil Miller.

Special gratitude, respect and love to my daughter, Michele Black, for her devotion and care giving; to my editor and cherished friend, Dennis Rystad, for his experience, and sense of humor during the writing of this book; to my copyeditor, Deborah Mink, for her special encouragement and patience; to my daughter-in-law, Elizabeth Fournier, for her design concept; to my stepson, Paul Fournier, Jr., for his patience and savvy, during occasional computer crises; and to my husband Paul Fournier—a true miracle in my life—whose inspiration, love and support has made this book possible.

Preface

To those of you who are interested in learning about Alzheimer's Disease, the following is the true story of my personal experience of the journey with my mother who was stricken. To those of you who are now dealing with a loved one's Alzheimer's Disease, you have my respect, and sympathy.

From my own experience, I suggest that if you suspect unusual changes in someone, document all behaviors and visit a doctor with this person, preferably a specialist in mind disorders or geriatrics. Diagnosis without concrete evidence is generally done through a process of elimination of other factors influencing changes in an individual. It will involve a complete physical and psychological work-up.

Once it can be assumed that Alzheimer's Disease is the cause of these changes, you will be able to handle the process if you arm yourself with as much information and education as you can obtain. Contact the Alzheimer's Association in your area, call 1-800-272-3900 or log on to www.alz.org to obtain additional information. This organization will be able to assist you through the changes you will experience in your loved one.

Don't isolate yourself. Keep in touch with family members, relatives and friends. Attend support groups. These interactive meetings provide support and respite from your care-giving responsibilities. You will receive valuable information, and the support group environment is an appropriate place to express your concerns.

Take the necessary action to maintain the individual in a safe environment. Shop around; look at all the possibilities. Some individuals may be able to remain at home for a time, cared for by the family until it becomes necessary for professionals to step in. Daycare services outside of the home provide temporary relief for family caregivers and give the stricken individual an organized and safe environment for recreation. At such facilities, he or she can interact and be as sociable as the stage of the illness permits. In time advanced stages of the disease will require that your loved one be placed in a care facility.

Seek legal counsel. You will have to make or participate in numerous legal decisions regarding the welfare of the individual in your care. In addition, to prove conclusively that the individual endured Alzheimer's Disease you may wish to order an autopsy. The authorization for this procedure can be arranged when you initiate establishing a conservatorship for the individual and must be in place before death occurs.

Staying focused and upbeat is helpful. Having a spiritual belief system, no matter what form it takes, may be helpful and supportive in keeping yourself together in mind, body and spirit. The disease is the most stressful on those who watch, wait and give care during its duration.

You are dealing with an adversary that will challenge you to the maximum. The situation is not going to improve, it is going to get worse. It is easy to feel overwhelmed and defeated. This is the reality of the disease process. There is no alternative, no reversal, no turn around. Alzheimer's Disease is degenerative, interminable and terminal. The duration of the disease process is from two to twenty years following prognosis.

Feeling angry, frightened, frustrated, embittered, helpless and sad are emotions to be expected. Obtaining information and making a plan of action will make the going easier. You can survive having to watch the disease's eroding affects on your loved one if you accept help and act realistically. Your attitude is the one element that will get you through this experience. You have the ability to decide how to look at the scenario unfolding in your life. I recommend you seek professional guidance while taking care of yourself in the process. The journey will be less traumatic. You will survive and go on from where you are.

I wish you well. I wish you as smooth a course as possible. May the light and warmth of the sun brighten any darkness on your side of the street.

Prayer for Strength

Dear God, give me the strength to cope
With this one day and not lose hope
Of pleasant vistas yet unseen
Tomorrows happy and serene

Give me the courage that I need
To banish every single seed
Of doubt, discouragement and fear
Blank misery and idle tear

Keep me aware, dear Lord, of you
The beautiful, the good and true
The power of love in which there's might
Enough to make things quite all right

Give me the breadth and depth of mind
To contemplate and seek and find
The certainty that for each man
You have a great and noble plan

Dear God, walk with me all this day
So I won't falter on the way
Transfer your strength and power to me
I ask in all humility

Helen Winter LaCaze

"The worst thing about this disease is that the person leaves you long before the person leaves you"

Robert Manne

Only Daughter   1

I n quiet moments of reverie, I can still see my mother Helen
  Winter LaCaze, and her husband Eddie dancing to a
throbbing jazz beat, laughing and recounting an evening of
adventure. I see their house at Christmas, trimmed in red lights
making the snowdrifts in the front yard pink. I can hear her
distinctive laugh across a crowded room as she emerges from the
party throng leading a conga. Mother always made a grand
entrance. No one who met her would soon forget her vivacity
and undeniable spirit—or believe one day she would enter and
leave rooms unnoticed.

Her story began in Saskatchewan, Canada. In the early 1900s,
the Canadian prairie was a frontier not unlike Minnesota and the
Dakotas a century earlier. Oscar and Jenny Winter and their three
sons were pioneers. Paul and Guy, the two oldest, found work
alongside their father on crews building a trans-Canadian
railroad. Hugh, who was much younger than his two brothers,
contracted a childhood illness, which left him completely deaf. He
spent his formative years in an institution for the hearing
impaired. Other workers and settlers formed a loose community
that grew to a village and then a town around the Winter family.
To honor his youngest son, Oscar named the town Hughton.

Hughton prospered and became a boomtown of its day,
largely due to Oscar's persistence and dedication to building a
railroad empire. He bought vast acreage of barren, flat land and
laid miles of beds, ties and tracks, weaving his way across the
prairie to spawn a healthy rail industry in other parts of the
province. His desire to create jobs and amass a fortune for his
family was short-lived, for he overextended his resources and

went bankrupt. With his resources wiped out, he and Jenny decided to return to their roots in the United States, to try and pick up the pieces of their life.

In another community some distance away, Christina Rinkes had been brought up to be unquestionably obedient to her German immigrant father. He, his wife and children had emigrated from Germany where he owned a small vineyard prior to the outbreak of World War I. Traveling by ship, steerage class, to freedom in Canada, they arrived and settled in a German community and observed their old country traditions.

The elder Rinkes was strict and unyielding when it came to his family. Christina's father demanded that she marry a wealthy widower when she was barely sixteen. The interested suitor was a farmer thirty years her senior. The union would offer Christina's father financial security for his floundering farm. In spite of Christina's protestations, her father began arrangements for the nuptials. Not wishing to be married to a man she didn't love, she ran away from home, never seeing her family again.

While working as a cook to support herself in Hughton, she met Paul Winter. They were married after a formal courtship, and settled down, a hopeful young couple on the Saskatchewan prairie. They immediately began raising a family. Mother once remarked to me that Grandma had conceived every year for the first several years of her marriage, a guarantee of at least one heir to carry on the name. The first three born were boys, and then on June 7, 1918, Helen Jane Winter was born. Paul and Christina were surprised but pleased by the addition of a girl, and later two more boys followed, making six children in all.

When Paul's father Oscar lost all of his resources, the younger Winter had to find new employment to support his pregnant wife and five young children. The struggling family lived on the outskirts of Hughton. The small dwelling in which they lived barely met their needs. The children had to share beds, and there was no indoor plumbing. Life was challenging and without luxuries. Years later, Grandma told my mother that going to the outhouse during a pregnancy in the dead of winter when the wind chill was fifty degrees below zero was not one of the pleasant memories of her early life in Canada.

Time passed on the prairie until fate stepped in on a winter evening. Paul and Christina had been invited to a barn dance at a distant farm. They both enjoyed dancing whenever the opportunity came. In spite of being pregnant with their sixth child, she was enthusiastic to attend but declined when Paul asked her to dance. He loved to dance and spent the evening square dancing to near exhaustion. Overheated from all the activity, he failed to cool off before starting home. Their horse-drawn sled slid easily over the snow-covered, wind-swept prairie, but he became chilled and fell ill, developing pneumonia. As he was lying struggling for breath in the small, Hughton hospital, Christina was in heavy labor with their sixth child. Paul died at the age of forty, never seeing his new son.

Christina was now a widow at age thirty-four with six children to feed and no income. As she had no place to turn except to her in-laws, she moved to Minneapolis, Minnesota in 1923. Though Oscar and Jenny were struggling to survive themselves, they welcomed her and the children into their modest home.

The first years following Paul's death were difficult for Christina. She had brought his body with her from Hughton for burial in the family plot at Lakewood Cemetery, a few blocks from her in-laws house. Mother told me that Grandma would go out to the cemetery weekly, kneel by his grave and weep. She was inconsolable and began to eat to fill the emptiness left by his passing. Over the years, she became morbidly overweight, a situation that later caused Mother concern and embarrassment. She was reluctant to bring friends home.

When Mother was born, Christina was pleased to have a daughter. "At last, I have a little lady to raise," she exclaimed with joy. But to my grandma's chagrin, Mother could have cared less about being a little lady. She chose to tag along with her brothers for the next eighteen years.

3

To her brothers too she was one of the boys and in spite of sibling squabbles and power struggles, Mother had enormous love for them. I believe Grandma's spirit of independence was passed on to Mother and developed in her as she grew up without a father. She had to keep up with her brothers, joining them in games and adventures, resulting in her becoming a tomboy. She considered herself equal to boys and insisted on the same rights as they had. This was a necessary posture in order to survive the traditional male dominance in her family.

Her oldest brother was Hugh, named after his deaf uncle. He was the most intellectual of the sons and developed an aptitude for mathematics and physics, graduating from high school when he was thirteen years old. He later earned the degree of *magna cum laude* and became one of a handful of nuclear physicists during the Cold War, retiring as a full colonel in the United States Army Air Corps. In his retirement from the service, he settled in New Mexico, one of his former tours of duty, and taught calculus at the University of Albuquerque.

Channing was next in the pecking order. Always a rebel, he ran away from home to ride the rails when he was in his teens and didn't return for several years. He became a brakeman and then a conductor for the railroad, carrying on the family tradition of working on the rails. As an adult he lived in Mankato, Minnesota. The small town environment suited him. He tolerated occasional trips to the Twin Cities but considered the metro area unsuitable for driving or living.

Vernon was the third son. He excelled in athletics, was a good student and socially popular in high school. He was forced to quit in his senior year and go to work during the Great Depression to help support the others at home. Graduating from night school, he worked his way up the corporate ladder by first loading boxcars for a local food store chain and later becoming vice president of warehousing and shipping. He excelled in his long career as a first class negotiator in labor and management relations.

Dale followed Mother and was a natural singer, a tenor. As the only artiste of the family, he also loved to sail and spent all his free time aboard a sailboat owned by a family friend in Forest Lake, Minnesota. It was said that the family lineage began by sailors who came over on the great ships. Dale was the only one of his generation who had sailing in his blood. During World War II he served in the United States Navy and was stationed aboard a ship in the Aleutian Islands.

Paul, named after his father who died as he was being born, was the baby of the family and by far the most mischievous child. On one occasion, Grandma told him to release a basket of garter snakes he had collected, and he chose a neighbors' yard for his deposit. The elderly lady living there was legally blind and couldn't discern between the sticks she was collecting and the wiggly critters crawling all over her backyard. As she picked up a snake, her scream could be heard all over the neighborhood. When Grandma found out about the incident, Paul had some explaining to do and an apology to make to the terrified woman. As he matured, he could spin a yarn better than anyone and became a first class salesman.

Very early in her life, Grandma taught her family that they were impoverished nobility. It was an apt description for the family. They had integrity and dignity, looked after each other and developed a closeness that served them best in the most challenging of times. Those who survived that bleak time in the history of the American economy knew the value of tenacity and a strong work ethic. This fierce determination to survive at all costs got them through the Great Depression of the 1930's. Grandma supported her children by working as a domestic. She was a hard worker and took pride in her work. On one occasion, a wealthy woman was giving her a list of chores to complete. Referring to Grandma as "Tina," she continued barking her demands.

"And when you are through in the kitchen, Tina, you can polish the woodwork."

"Yes, Madam," my grandma responded as she straightened up from scrubbing the floor.

"I want a bright finish on the woodwork. Understood, Tina?"

Grandma had had enough of the unwanted nickname, and at that moment straightened all four feet ten inches of herself to look directly into the offensive woman's eyes. "Mrs. Winter to you, Madam!"

Those who hired her had great respect for her dignity and perseverance. Mother's grandparents, in spite of the lack of resources, taught their grandchildren the value of diligence and honesty. All through the Depression years, the Winter siblings grew strong and resourceful, resulting in a fierce independence that they all carried the rest of their lives.

My uncle Paul once shared a story with me about Mother. In 1928, at the age of eight, my uncle Dale found a golf club and ball and decided to try them. He took the items to the boulevard green near the curb in front of the house. He was small for his age, but he was determined to hit the ball even though the club handle was tucked under his chin.

Mother came along and decided she wanted to try a shot. An argument ensued. "Helen, girls don't hit golf balls," Dale insisted, waving his older sister aside as he prepared to swing the club. Mother was not so easily dismissed.

"Oh yeah, says who? I'm two years older and a lot taller than you, Dale!"

Dale knew he could never win an argument from Mother. He finally relented saying, "Ok for you! Here, take the club! Girls!" She took a couple of practice swings as Dale stood behind her, determined to guide his older sister. Mother set up the ball and swung with all her might. On the follow-through the club head caught Dale right above the eye. She heard a loud scream, turned around and discovered Dale on the ground, covered with blood. He looked like he had been to the slaughterhouse.

Unflappable, Mother helped her little brother up, calmly walked him home and kept repeating, "I'm sorry, Dale. It was an accident, honest! It isn't so bad, really!" Uncle Paul concluded his story—"Dale wore the scar to his grave and Helen never did learn to play golf."

One Christmas, Grandma didn't have enough money to buy the children gifts. Money was scarce and she could barely put food on the table. Feeling hopeless, she was in a distracted state when Mother ran into the room saying, "Ma, come quick, come and see out the window!" Pulling back the curtain, Grandma noticed a long, black limousine parked on the street. A uniformed driver was reaching into the trunk and pulling out some brightly wrapped presents, which he piled alongside the curb. When he finished, he picked up the pile, precariously balancing them as he made his way up to the front porch. Setting down the colorful packages, he rang the bell. Grandma opened the door at once.

"Mrs. Winter?"

"Yes?"

For a moment, the driver tipped his hat and smiled at Grandma. "My employer wishes to remain anonymous, but she would like to wish you and your children a 'Merry Christmas!' Please accept these as a token of her gratitude and respect."

Grandma was not ready for a Santa Claus in jodhpurs, nor the gifts he brought, but with her usual grace she responded, "Thank you so much. Please extend holiday greetings to your employer!"

The driver picked up the packages and brought them into the front parlor. By now, all the Winter kids were standing by, observing him as he piled the gifts in the middle of the room. When he had finished his errand, he turned to Grandma and the children, clicked his heels together, bowed gallantly and smiled, uttering a hearty, "Good night, madam!"

Mother said that was one Christmas she never forgot.

Growing up in the City of Lakes, Mother became a young tadpole. A typical summer day in the life of the Winter kids was to leave the house early in the morning with a packed lunch and head for Calhoun Lake which was a few blocks away. Mother and her two younger brothers Dale and Paul would swim across the lake, each watching out for the other. She became an accomplished swimmer. Her body was flexible and supple and she had above average endurance and strength. She was fit through all the conditioning that comes from exercise and had an outstanding figure.

As agile as she was, she still sustained some minor injuries in her tomboy youth. She enjoyed climbing a tree in the backyard of the Winter home. Hanging from one of the branches by her knees, Mother pretended to be a circus aerialist. Grandma often harped on the dangers of hi-jinks too high off the ground, but her warnings fell on deaf ears. Mother continued hanging by her knees purposely swinging back and forth because she enjoyed it, as well as in defiance of her mother. One afternoon as she was swinging upside down, she slipped, fell to the ground and was knocked unconscious. Moments later she came to, stood up, and brushed herself off. She never mentioned the fall to Grandma and undaunted, continued to climb trees and swing by her knees whenever a branch beckoned.

Of Grandma's children, Mother was the only child who enjoyed sliding down the banister from the second floor to the vestibule just inside the front door of the house. She loved sailing down the smooth surface, especially with her hands free. Once again, Grandma warned her that it was dangerous and highly unladylike. Mother scoffed at caution and with boundless enthusiasm continued to sail down the stairs behind Grandma's back. True, she took a few bumps and lumps, but she never reported them.

Mother's fearless brothers took chances too, and as she was able to keep up with their various shenanigans, she earned their respect. She was, after all, their only sister, and she was tomboy tough.

In addition to Mother's love of water, she enjoyed biking, bowling, canoeing, and tennis. As she grew older, she could put in a full day at work and still have enough energy to do something interesting and challenging with her free time.

She loved the city lakes. Being able to walk or ride on her bicycle around them gave her a sense of peace and belonging in the great outdoors. She enjoyed them in all seasons, and during the frigid winter common in Minnesota, she enjoyed feeding the wildlife. She saved stale bread and brought it in a plastic bag to distribute amongst her feathered friends, the wild geese and ducks that hung out along the shore of Lake of the Isles. Their quacking seemed to acknowledge that she was a friend. Sitting on a convenient wooden bench, she also found joy and humor in watching the parade of people as they passed her way.

As the years went by, and circumstances separated the Winter siblings geographically, the special bond that had developed in their childhood remained intact. They wrote, telephoned and visited each other and their families whenever possible. Time and distance could not erase the pride and respect they had developed, a family bond based not only on a chance of birth but on the shared experience of surviving and prospering in spite of poverty. The Winters were a combined force of integrity and resiliency. Mother carried those qualities for the rest of her life.

Unbridled Enthusiasm   2

My earliest recollection of my mother was her warm smile, her beautiful teeth and her vivacious personality. I remember her oval face fringed by dark curly bangs and dominated by snappy green eyes with brown specks. Mother had a figure that was movie-star gorgeous. She tried to emulate her favorite actress Joan Crawford. To me she was prettier. She was the most beautiful lady in the world!

Mother did not always follow convention but consistently tried to do what was right or best for us. Divorce in those days was a drastic step. Often divorcees were thought of as less than morally virtuous for having failed at marriage. Mother and my father, John Stoddart, were two very different individuals. Living together during the first few months of marriage only proved how incompatible they were. He was insecure and possessive, while Mother was a free spirit, impossible to pin down.

They both worked in the advertising department at Gambles. My father was a commercial artist and Mother wrote copy. One day Mother felt ill and decided to stay home. When my father returned home that evening he flew into a jealous rage over an imagined affair involving Mother and an unknown party. During their altercation, he grabbed Mother around the neck and began choking her. She managed to free herself and convinced him to calm down.

Mother, pregnant and fearing for her safety, left him the first opportunity she had. For her to continue living with such an unstable person was unthinkable. She filed for divorce citing irrevocable differences and got sole custody of me. Mother wiped the slate clean, never looking back. She never saw my father again and the court ordered him to stay away from me.

After the divorce Mother devoted the next eighteen years to raising me as a single parent. She faced many challenges because there weren't as many women who were single parents in the 1940s as there are today. She worked full time, supporting Grandma, herself and me. Grandma had been left without the benefit of social security or pension and was dependent on my mother for a home. She lived with us and took care of me while Mother worked. Mother was enterprising and never complained. She would return from a full day of work, tired as she was, recharge her batteries and spend quality time with me. These activities included field trips to the zoo or picnics by a lake. But my favorite pastime was hearing Mother's stories or learning to draw by watching her.

In the early forties Mother continued working in advertising as a copywriter. McCann-Erickson in Minneapolis hired her to join the creative group working on the Pillsbury account. She loved words and enjoyed stirring them up like a cake mix.

She had a reputation for coming up with outrageous ideas for new ad campaigns, and she took enormous creative risks to juice up the material she was working on.

In a creative meeting on one occasion, the big brass of the local agency including the head account executive from the New York office gathered around a conference table to hear the presentation for a new cake product. As Mother told it, "There they sat like stiff soldiers waiting for their orders as they drank coffee and smoked cigarettes, each trying to impress the other with advertising lingo and forced rhetoric."

The creative team assembled and Mother chanted the pitch.

Patty cake, patty cake, baker's man
Pillsbury bakes it as good as you can.
Mix it, stir it, fold it in a bowl
You'll love this cake, 'cause it really has soul!

As she chanted her parody of the familiar children's rhyme, she danced around the table, snapping her fingers and clapping like a child, singing.

When she finished, there was silence in the boardroom. The creative group sat motionless, eyes lowered, waiting for the ax to fall. Mother's supervisor was visibly shaken.

Then one by one the big brass began to applaud. They loved her idea. George Sparling, Mother's boss, was noticeably relieved. After the meeting had wrapped however, George pulled her aside and suggested, "In the future Helen, ideas should be approved by me before the pitch." Mother's jingle was never heard over the airwaves because Pillsbury was a conservative client at the time. Later, the agency lost the account, but not due to Mother's verve.

Working as a secretary was another way she supported us, but her true passion was creative writing. Her material was expressive and personal. Her ability to create great stories was her hallmark and as she matured, the more she wrote the better her writing got.

Mother would regale me with her poems and stories and they filled me with wonder and curiosity. Our particular favorites were *Winnie the Pooh* and *The House at Pooh Corner* by A. A. Milne. Not only would Mother create voices for the characters, she would make up tunes to match the author's words and sing them to me. Listening raptly, I lost track of the time.

Mother told me years later that, like many other children, I had an imaginary brother. His name was Tommy, and she interacted with him as well. When I grew tired of him, she claimed Tommy enlisted in the army and he went off to boot camp somewhere in Oklahoma! Sad to say, I don't remember Tommy at all.

Mother also created a great character named Hoibie, a mountain lion that went everywhere with us, especially when we rode the bus. We would climb aboard, and Mother would drop the fare in the box. We walked down the aisle chatting with Hoibie as we looked for a seat. Mother became Hoibie's voice, deepening her own, until it became a gravelly growl.

"Hey, Hoibie, which side of the bus do you want to sit on?" She'd look up at the imagined playmate as he walked on his hind legs, following us up the aisle.

He'd speak through Mother, "Oh, shucks, I don't know. I hate decisions!"

Sometimes we would find a row of seats at the back of the bus, enough space to allow all three of us to sit. Passengers' eyes would widen. Some would change seats moving to a more comfortable distance as Mother continued to converse with an empty space occupied by a giant, invisible cat.

Occasionally while waiting for a bus Mother would lose all patience with me. It would be the dead of winter, freezing cold, snow falling, the wind whipping down the street and I would not get on a city bus that wasn't smiling.

"Honey, is that one smiling?"

Only I knew how to identify a bus with a welcoming face. "No, can't you see?"

Mother would peer through the blinding snow, hoping for a break. "Are you sure?"

"Mooothhher!"

Sometimes two and three buses would stop but I would refuse to get on until one pulled up with a smiley expression. Mother waited patiently, never wanting to fuss about my obvious determination. "What about this one?"

When at last a bus came along that was acceptable to me, she was visibly relieved to step out of the bone-chilling cold into the inviting warmth and be on our way.

One of Mother's greatest accomplishments took place when I turned ten. She wanted to buy me my first bicycle, an item she could ill afford. She put in extra hours at the office in order to save up enough money to purchase the bike. The day it was ready for pick-up, instead of having it delivered she rode it home, singing all the way. The bright sheen of the new blue bike must have delighted her because she was laughing. When I saw her ride up to the back of the house, I eagerly ran out to meet her by the garage.

"Oh, Christine! Isn't it a beauty?" She got off for only a moment, running her fingers over its shiny finish and then insisted on breaking it in for me! I will always remember the sight of her perching on that glistening two-wheeler, peddling around and around the block until she had had enough.

Her enthusiasm was infectious and even the neighbors commented about Mother's pleasure with her new toy. It took a couple of weeks for me to get comfortable riding my new bike. Mother was patient and held on to the back as I learned how to balance on the two-wheeler. One day when she was guiding me she gently let go and I was on my own, half way down the block before suddenly realizing it. I turned and saw her watching me, an enormous smile on her face.

From the time I was a toddler, she always had me in tow, and as a result I developed a love for walking from my earliest years. We walked everywhere; to church, to the movies, to visit friends, to and around the lakes near our neighborhood, and to the grocery store once a week where we would shop and then take a cab home.

I loved tree shopping at Christmas. We did this close to the apartment, because we knew we would have to carry our selection home. Only once did a kind stranger offer to tie the tree to the top of his car and drive us home. Mother accepted graciously.

At other times we would lift the tree, each taking an end, and proceed on our merry way, trudging through freshly fallen snow as the light from the street lamps provided a magic glow to the evening. Laughing, our breath puffing out and fogging the air ahead of us, we would take breaks along the way, dropping the tree and sitting down on a nearby step to rest. Still cold but happy, we would resume our mission, enjoying our success the rest of the way home.

Within a few minutes, the tree was secured upright in a water-filled stand. We gradually warmed up sipping hot cocoa and admiring our selection. The stately tree stood in the middle of our living room, and as the warm dry air encircled it, the fragrance of fresh-cut evergreen filled the apartment. Eventually its branches began to relax and drop, creating the impression of a much grander acquisition.

To get around when I was a child, we depended on the city bus or the streetcar that ran on rails. The Como-Harriet streetcar was my favorite mode of transportation. I loved the way it would sway and squeal down the tracks. The conductor pulled the cord to ring the bell as a signal at stops. Once passengers were safely discharged or boarded, the big yellow car rattled on its way, taking us from home to downtown Minneapolis, to the dentist in Morningside, to the Como Zoo in St. Paul, or sometimes to the picnic grounds at Lake Harriet.

Going on a picnic to the lake was one of my most treasured activities with Mother. On these outings she would make an adventure of it, carrying all the picnic supplies in a large basket. Once in the park, we would collect wood, and she would make a small fire. We found long skinny sticks to spear wieners and marshmallows that we roasted over the fire. The hot dogs would split and the juice would pop as it hit the fire, filling our noses with mouthwatering aromas. The marshmallows would turn tan, puff out and sometimes catch fire, and we'd blow them out to find white dripping out of the charred shell.

When we finished eating, I would sit on a swing, Mother pushing me higher and higher until I yelled, "Stop!" The slides intimidated me and after my obvious reluctance to climb the high steps to the top, Mother would go first, assuring me that it was easy as pie. I had no choice but to follow suit, and once I did it, Mother couldn't get me to stop. Tired and spent from all the fresh lake air, we would return home by the clanging and rattling streetcar, having had a marvelous day.

Relatives drove us to family events. We would be invited to my Uncle Vernon's house where Aunt Frances would prepare delightful dinners on Sundays and holidays.

Following World War II, khaki green was the most widely used color, and I remember my uncle Vernon picking us up in a khaki green car. Traveling by car was a hideous experience. I would get motion sick. I developed a subconscious association of the color green with being nauseated. No matter how Mother tried to dissuade me from hating automobiles, I wanted no part of them. It took me dozens of car rides to overcome my distaste for motoring and the color green.

Walking however was never distasteful and it was a habitual pleasure my mother cultivated in me as a healthy and necessary activity. I think my love of moving through space started with walking, then skipping and hopping, and childishly twirling around the living room.

Mother loved moving too. When a date would escort her out for an evening, she'd suggest dancing. She would dance every dance and usually leave her date exhausted and sitting one out while she danced with others as fast as they approached her.

Later at home she regaled me with her dance experiences, "He moved like Fred Astaire, twirling me until I was dizzy!" She was glowing from all the activity.

"Really, Mom?" I sat transfixed as she demonstrated how her date placed his arm around her waist and then guided her with his free hand. There was always a colorful account of each partner.

"Then this big guy with three left feet cut in and all but destroyed my two!"

"How did you get out of that one?" By now I was glued to the demonstration before me.

"Another spotted my predicament, took over and taught me a dance called the cha-cha."

I was an avid listener and watched, spellbound, as Mother showed me the latest steps.

Her love of dance spilled over into me. She saw that I had a gift for mimicry too, and when I was five she enrolled me in a basic dance class for very young children offered at MacPhail Center For The Arts in downtown Minneapolis.

The teacher was very heavy set and seemed to have a limited knowledge of dance. She would waddle across the floor and as the tempo accelerated, she attempted to keep time, gliding tenuously. Generous thighs wiggling, she finished with a pose, looking more like a Disney animated character than a famous ballerina like Anna Pavlova.

For my first recital we performed a dance called "The Lollipop Parade." We had to carry giant lollipops made from cardboard on stands. While even at five I had strong instincts toward dance movement, Mother knew I was too young for serious training. She waited two years before enrolling me in more disciplined work. When I was seven and my bones were stronger and my feet could withstand classic ballet training, she enrolled me in a Russian Ballet class.

In the interim between my early dance class experience and my enrollment in Russian Ballet training, Mother's love for dancing continued. I remember on one occasion she was walking through the backyard and accidentally stepped on a bee. She was severely stung and her foot swelled to twice its normal size. Undaunted, she did not cancel her date for the evening, as her escort was a favorite beau. I can still see her hobbling out of the house, hanging on his arm, a trail of giggles etching the sky of that tepid summer evening. The joy and anticipation of dancing overcame the pain in her puffy foot.

Occasionally as a child I would become anxious when Mother wasn't in view. Once, I approached our cellar from an outside yard door, having seen her disappear into the basement to do some laundry. A tapping sound drew me to listen at the basement door. Cautiously I opened the door and peeked inside, my eyes adjusting to the dim light. "Tap-clickity-tap-clickity." Mother was tap dancing to the sound and rhythm of the washing machine's agitation. Her patent-leather shoes shone as she tapped and spun, her tempo accelerating in a whirl of giddy enthusiasm. She had never had a tap lesson in her life, but somehow had acquired the skill by watching tappers in movie musicals. In her mind, she became another favorite actress of the time, perhaps Eleanor Powell incarnate, at least on the days she washed.

During my seventh year, Mother took me to the classic film *The Red Shoes*. From the moment I saw Moira Shearer, the red-haired ballerina of the movie, I knew I wanted to dance just like her. Hypnotized, I watched her handsome partner Robert Helpmann lift her into the air. I was hooked; dancing was my destiny. Mother knew it too. In the years that followed she paid for after-school ballet lessons twice a week from an accomplished teacher.

His name was Victor Stengal, a Polish displaced person, who in his youth had soloed in Kiev and Moscow. He was sponsored by a local dance school owner, Mr. Kugler, who realized the need for good, classic training in the Upper Midwest. He moved Mr. Stengal and his entire family to Minneapolis and set him up in his own school to teach classic Russian ballet.

I was fortunate to be among Mr. Stengal's first American students, and the training was excellent. The lessons were costly, given Mother's tight budget, but she realized that my talent couldn't be denied. I needed a good teacher, and Mr. Stengal was that teacher. In broken English he'd often comment, "American girls aren't serious about ballet!" He tapped a large cane on the floor in time to the musical accompaniment from a careworn upright piano stashed in the corner of the long studio, pounded on by a bone-thin, squinty-eyed maiden lady.

Large mirrors covered the wall opposite the bar where we all lined up during class. We began each class with strenuous warm-ups, stretching and pulling and asking our bodies to do the impossible, and all the while Victor would walk down the line of young girls, correcting turn-outs, straightening backs and muttering expletives in a mixture of English, Polish and Russian. I had to learn to decipher the language code.

I was ecstatic when Mother would stop in after her workday and observe class from the chairs at the sidelines, and I worked even harder when she was in attendance, feeling proud that she had come to watch me.

Mother bought me all the necessary supplies in order to attend class: soft ballet slippers, tights and leotards. And when the time came and I was physically developed enough, I was fitted for toe shoes! How she managed to afford and supply me with the necessities for dance training I will never know, but she did it unselfishly. All through my formative years, Mother stood back, proud and encouraging. She was patient and enthusiastic as her dedicated daughter danced her way through blistered and bleeding toes, sweaty leotards and pre-teen chubbiness.

Mother had several chances to marry during my childhood years. She was discerning about whom she dated and often included me in outings with her favorite escorts. Sometimes her date would take us to the movies, to the park or out to dinner. Each was a special treat. If she began dating a man and he showed little or no interest in me, he was soon discarded.

One gentleman she saw regularly turned out to be a favorite of mine. Amehl, a former professional dancer, was movie-star handsome. He adored Mother and wanted to marry her in spite of the differences in their religious upbringing. She would not adopt his faith and refused to ask him to give up his. Instead, she ended the relationship, leaving him heartbroken and herself alone once more. I was sad to see their relationship cease, as he had been very loving toward Mother and accepting of me.

When I was thirteen, Mother introduced me to Donald Stewart, who was charming, handsome and socially adept. He came from a fine Scottish family and his affectionate demeanor, pleasant personality and impeccable manners won Mother's heart. After a brief courtship, they decided to marry.

Donald was a salesman who sold air freshener products to industry. He appeared successful during their first year of marriage, but as time passed he was unable to develop and sustain his client base and as a result lost his job. Mother became the sole breadwinner. When Donald wasn't sleeping the day away, he was at the local watering hole, spending money that should have been used for household expenses, and soon creditors were calling with threats.

However, the final straw occurred when my grandma Christina was dying, and everyone in the family was taking a turn at vigil. Donald, seeing that Mother was wearing down, volunteered to take her place one evening, making the trip to the nursing home several miles away. Exhausted, she fell into a deep sleep and in the morning, learned that her mother had died during the night.

When she questioned Donald about Christina's last moments, he gave a detailed account of her death. Later she found out from another member of the family that Donald was in a bar when my grandma died, which was unforgivable in Mother's eyes. This betrayal along with his irresponsibility and unwillingness to provide for the family was too much for her. She asked him to leave and subsequently hired a lawyer and divorced him. Back on her own, she gradually paid off creditors and re-established her independent lifestyle.

Mother wasn't interested in dating. After her second divorce and subsequent financial ruin, she had little use for men. She had been burned and preferred to live her life without a partner. She determined that she could take care of herself and me better than any man who might come along would.

For the next three years, we shared an apartment we had rented after the Donald fiasco. We were two women facing the world together.

It was during this period that Mother began writing articles pertaining to life with an adolescent. She had a striking and articulate way of describing the mind of a teenager. In the fifties, when I was going to high school, I readily fueled her imaginative fire. The poems and essays she wrote became a flowing commentary on the adventures of a single mom raising a teenage daughter. Often these writings aided her in deciding how to handle a situation as it arose.

In the spring of 1958 she wrote:

To Chris with Tolerance and Love

Mother, may I go out tonight?
A new boy's asked for a date
I never thought he'd ask, but he has
And, Mother we won't be late.
Oh, how could I be so lucky?
He's not only cute, he's cool
He's a letter man, on the honor roll
The neatest boy in school.
He is absolutely darling
I flipped when he gave me the eye
He smiled at me in the hall one day and
I honestly thought I'd die.
His haircut is really the most
He's tall and his eyes are blue
And all of the girls are crazy for him
He drives a convertible too.

Yes, you may go out, sweet daughter
Yes, you may go out with him
Such a paragon should not be refused
But whatever happened to Jim?
Last week Jim was first on your list

Without doubt, a walking dream
So completely, so utterly, darling
His telephone calls made you scream.

Oh, Mother, you really are square
You don't understand that's all
Jim's all right as a friend but we're finished
Just wait till you see this boy, Paul.
Oh, Mother, I just had a thought
A most overwhelming one yet
There are thousands, no millions of darling boys
In the world that I've never met.

At times, she would write more philosophically about her challenges. She expressed her feelings in different forms developing a poem, a prayer, or an essay to clarify her thoughts. At other times she wrote with engaging humor and wisdom.

In 1960 she wrote:

Just One Day

Although your sky is full of rain
Don't throw yourself beneath a train
Don't scream and shake your fist at fate
And view the world with fear and hate
'Tis true that anyone can cope
With just one day, while gripping hope
One day, that's all, so very brief
Can hold a minimum of grief
Mayhap your cup is brimming sorrow
But why not wait and cry tomorrow?

Her writing clearly expressed the moment in which she was engaged. Sifting through her thoughts and then releasing them on paper was Mother's unique way of sharing what was going on with her at a particular time.

Eddie LaCaze 3

O ur lives changed when Mother met Edward Herman LaCaze. Mutual friends insisted they get together and arranged a blind date. Naturally, Mother was wary about going out with someone she didn't know, but Edward came highly recommended. Eddie, or 'Frenchie,' a nickname he was given by his fellow lodge brothers, was a widower in his mid-fifties, owned his own business, a painting/decorating company, and was an active Freemason and member of Zuhrah Shrine Temple.

Eddie had been born in New Orleans and raised by his mother who worked as a domestic after his father deserted them. She remarried and together, she and her second husband Bill Miller provided a stable environment for Eddie. He grew up with a disarmingly direct manner and his integrity was unquestionable. He was mature and worldly, possessing the right mix of street smarts and gentlemanly acumen.

Eddie had married for the first time when he was in his late thirties and after fifteen years he was left a widower by the death of his wife. Eddie was lonely and in need of companionship and for two years continued to live in the house they had shared, with only his Irish Terrier Tuzy to fill the void.

When Eddie came into Mother's life we were living in Dinkytown, a student area near the University of Minnesota campus. I was attending college there and involved in my own world, taking courses in theatre and dance. We shared a little apartment on campus from which I could walk to classes every day and Mother could commute to her job by bus. It was a convenient arrangement for both of us, as well as a lot of fun, and we were as involved in each other's worlds as we always had been.

Mother and Eddie's first date was a sit-down dinner for eight guests at his home. He prepared the meal and served it himself. Mother was impressed with his grace, humor and values.

The first time I met Eddie, he had come to pick up Mother for a date. The buzzer sounded, and as I opened the door I was not prepared for the vision of *savoir faire* that radiated from the other side of the threshold. There stood a gentleman so immaculately groomed, so self-assured, so finely dressed, he took my breath away. He smelled of Old Spice that accented his clean-shaved face, sported a dapper pencil-thin mustache and had gray hair at his temples. The soft olive green velvet fedora with a snazzy little brush along the side of the brim only added to his splendor, and he was wearing a camel's hair coat. He held matching leather gloves in one hand. In the other, he held a leash attached to a large, orange fuzzy dog with a big smile and pointy ears that sat politely waiting for permission to move. My mouth must have gaped open but Eddie took it all in his stride.

"Hello," I managed to stammer as I shifted from one foot to the other.

"Good evening, you must be Chris. I am here for Helen." By now the pleasant aroma of his after-shave had invaded my senses, and I forgot my manners entirely until I realized that the man was overheating in the hall in his winter outerwear.

"Oh, please come in, Eddie. I'll let Mom know you're here." Eddie carefully wiped his snow-covered rubbers on the braided doormat, and then he and his fuzzy orange companion stepped carefully inside. I backed away from this class act and his equally gentrified canine, and went to find Mother who was, at this point, behaving like a teenage girl as she nervously applied the last touches of makeup.

"Mom, he's here!"

"Oooooh, I'm so nervous! How do I look?" Mother had borrowed one of my dresses and looked fabulous. The emerald green of the fabric brought out the brown in her eyes and they glistened with excitement.

This became a familiar scenario. For over a month, they courted and cooed like a couple of lovebirds. When they weren't working, they were together. They went to dances, parties, and events. Eddie loved to cook romantic dinners for the two of them at his home. Obviously they were falling in love.

I was surprised by the speed of their courtship, but my concerns gave way when I observed Mother's obvious happiness with Eddie.

One day, two months after they had started dating, she told me that Eddie proposed. She said that at that moment she was so taken aback, she stammered at Eddie.

"Don't you want to know about my past? You know nothing about me!"

Eddie took her hands firmly in his and said gently, "Helen, I know all I need to know!"

"But my past."

"We all have them! Please do me the honor of marrying me."

Much to my delight, they were married three months later on April 22, 1961 in a small ceremony. The Reverend George Butters, a fellow Mason, presided. Only the immediate family and a few close friends attended. I observed a great celebration, the joining of two dear souls. Within a month, they bought a new house in a new community and settled in.

When I came home from college on the weekends, I would do all the necessary catching up that students require. I did my loads of laundry, grabbed as much sleep as possible and ate marvelous meals. Mother prepared them but Eddie supervised. He was a great chef. He taught Mother to make everything from

New Orleans style red beans and rice to biscuits from scratch, the way his mother had taught him.

Mother became quite a cook in her own right. We lived what I imagined a traditional family life was. Eddie was thrilled to have a daughter, as he and his late wife had never had children. I was pleased to have a dad. Eddie filled the void left by Mother's early divorce from my father. Mother was happy, and that made everything right.

Mother enjoyed Eddie's activities in Freemasonry. In addition, he was an active member of Zuhrah Temple that hosted big events. Mother and Eddie never missed an opportunity to party. When it came to social dancing they hardly ever sat one out. Together they were equally adept at dancing to grand orchestras playing the standards as to a five-piece combo blasting good Dixieland jazz. Often, in the wee hours of Sunday morning, I would wake up with a start at the sounds of their laughter and talking as they returned home. Once awake, I would join them in the living room where they regaled me with details of the party.

They took turns describing their antics, enjoying a couple of drinks while I sipped ginger ale. In great detail, Eddie described Mother's solo dancing and singing as she drew a large crowd around her. She would lift her skirt, showing her fabulous legs, shimmy to a drum riff and accent her nimble moves with a bump and grind. The crowd went wild.

Eddie stood back captivated by Mother as she worked the audience. To my knowledge, he was never jealous in all the years they were together. He was proud of her and loved all the attention she received. His merriment at their recital of Mother's antics was infectious and his love for her was obvious. They developed the reputation of being leaders of the party pack. As the sun was coming up, the stories and laughter ran down and we retired for some much-needed sleep.

For my twentieth birthday, Mother and Eddie threw a party for me and invited all the performers of the University of Minnesota *Showboat* cast, of which I was a part.

Halfway through an evening of Italian spaghetti and flowing gin and tonic, Mother decided to dance to banjo music provided by cast members. As the musicians began plunking out a spirited tune, Mother merrily danced her way through the sizeable crowd of party guests.

The next morning, she was doing her best to avoid eye contact with anything edible. Noticing her apparent discomfort I joked that it was one thing to do a tabletop solo, but asked, "Did everyone have to end the evening knowing the color of your panties?"

Mother laughed it off saying, "Well, after all dear, red is my signature color!" In spite of her hangover, Mother's *joie de vivre* left me smiling and proud that my mother wasn't a square.

Mother never missed any of my shows if she could help it. She attended recitals, high school plays, and local community theatre productions. Later, she came to New York to see her only progeny's success dancing on a Broadway stage.

Her enthusiasm extended to live theatre and to movies as well. I heard her laughter in many auditoriums through the years. Her laugh, unique and hard to forget, was a cross between a bellow and a loud cackle. The sound would start low then grow in intensity, full and heartfelt, until it was ricocheting off the walls of the theatre. Mother's voice was so unusual that heads would turn and a murmur would glide through the audience. When I was younger and less sure of myself, I would slide down in my seat, embarrassed, hoping that no one had seen me with her.

I once watched her with her brother Channing attending a film together. It was an outrageous comedy and Mother and her brother became involved in the action, hitting each other while in the throes of their hilarity. This tendency to lose control when amused must run in the family genes because it seems to have been passed on to me.

One of my early career engagements was appearing in the *How To Succeed In Business Without Really Trying* national tour that played in Minneapolis and St. Paul. Mother and Eddie not only attended many of the run's performances, they sat front row center and invited groups of friends to join them. They were obviously proud of me and wanted to share my triumph of "small town girl makes good" with their best pals.

Seeing all those wonderfully supportive and familiar faces in the first few rows of the orchestra section choked me up and brought goose bumps. I was thrilled to be playing my hometown.

Local skeptics had predicted I would fail in New York City and come home with my tail between my legs. They also attended and sat in the front row of the theatre. During the big dance number in the second act, I spotted them and they were cheering. When I was struggling to survive in order to stay in New York, Eddie had said, "Chris, when you're having a hard time no one wants to buy you as much as a hamburger, but when you make it, they all will want to buy you steak!" I never forgot his observation.

During the show's engagement, Mother and Eddie threw a cast party at their home in the suburbs. The New York-based cast members, in the hinterlands without transportation, resorted to taxi service. Whole fleets of cabs kept arriving and departing throughout the evening and into the wee hours.

Some musicians brought instruments and started jamming. You can guess who ended up in the middle of the group. Mother danced the night away with stagehands, wardrobe people, and of course, the male dancers known as "gypsies."

I honestly think if Mother had not been ensconced in her life with Eddie, she might have stowed away on the cast train, joining us for the rest of the tour as we made our way across the country. The morning we departed the Twin Cities, I was never sure if Mother was crying because she was sad to see me go or because we were leaving without her.

Some years after that first tour I won a chorus spot in the original *Sweet Charity* starring Gwen Verdon, directed and choreographed by Bob Fosse. One New Year's weekend Mother arrived in Detroit on a whim where we were going through the rigors of what is known as an "out-of-town tryout." Her timing was impeccable. She could come to a special party that the producers Robert Fryer, Lawrence Carr, Joseph and Sylvia Harris, and playwright Neil Simon threw for the company in an enormous ballroom.

As the walls shook and the cast reveled, Mother ended up in a conga line led by Bob Fosse, which wound around the ballroom. Later, a character actress from the cast who ended up on Rowan and Martin's *Laugh-In*, and internationally acclaimed *Sesame Street*, comedienne Ruth Buzzi, latched on to Mother. Together they crawled under tables and gleefully moved them across the dance floor, startling several on-lookers.

The party continued into the wee hours of New Year's morning, but I finally managed to drag Mother out of the ballroom and back to the hotel.

I woke up the next day with my first hangover and had to face a brush-up rehearsal and two shows with the shakes. Mother plied me with black coffee and suggested, "Chris, if you could manage to throw up you'll definitely feel better!" I groaned at the mere thought of throwing up, but I was listening to the voice of experience.

The irony was that Mother, who partied long and hard, felt great the next day and was once again ready to take on the world. I on the other hand had to go on for the understudy who understudied the stand-by for Miss Verdon. She was out ill and so the line and pecking order, of understudies and swing dancers, moved up as we faced the two shows without the star attraction. Two full bottles of club soda later, I vowed never to have a hangover again.

Mother saw one performance of the show, but the highlight of her visit was to watch Mr. Fosse create one of the numbers being added, "Rhythm of Life." Mother sat at the back of the dark theatre watching Bob create staging to the music we had previously rehearsed vocally for two weeks in Philadelphia.

Later Sunday, after rehearsal, she grabbed my arm and gushed, "What a privilege it was watching Fosse put you through your paces. You imitated everything he did exactly like him." I always cherished her comments.

Mother saw *Sweet Charity* again in New York at the Palace Theatre a year after it opened, and she was just as enthusiastic. She whooped and applauded from her seat whenever I appeared on stage, and her reactions created a ripple effect throughout the audience.

"You know Mom, I think the management of the theatre should pay you to attend the show every night and start a chain reaction," I told her.

She responded with a nod and a giggle. "Ah ha, I understand. I'd be a paid laugher. I'm ready!"

No matter what audience she was in, I always knew where she was seated. There was no escaping that laugh!

One of my favorite moments with Mother took place years later on the opening night of *Sweet Charity* at the former Chimera Theatre in downtown St. Paul. I was doing the lead in the show, playing Charity Hope Valentine.

There is a moment during the second act of a musical known as the ten-thirty spot, a musical number placed strategically to wake up those napping.

During the introduction to "I'm a Brass Band," the music swells and you sense a big number is about to begin. As the number took off, a very familiar voice rang out of the audience: "Give 'em hell, Chris!" Mother had very noticeably enhanced the performance's ten-thirty spot. Anyone still dozing must have been deaf.

Most cherished of all my memories of Mother's unbridled enthusiasm was the time in downtown Chicago when she led a drum and bugle corps down Wacker Drive at high noon. She and Eddie were attending a national convention of Shriners. They were on the curb watching the parade of nobles going by when Mother suddenly stepped off the curb in time to the beat, walked into the middle of the avenue, and took the baton from the bandleader. When he realized it was Helen LaCaze, he bowed, stepped aside and motioned her to take his place as the leader of the band. He then fell into line following her down the street. The startled onlookers began to applaud and those musicians who were not tooting on their instruments at that moment, yelled "It's Helen LaCaze" when they realized Frenchie's lady was their leader. Chicago's finest blew their whistles, stomped to the beat, and sent up a round of enthusiastic cheers. The people crowding the sidewalks at that moment were treated to the sight of an incredible lady clad in red, leading a colorful contingent of Shriners. They would surely remember that parade for a long time to come.

Mother and Eddie were soul mates in the truest sense. Their personalities, needs and philosophies were compatible, and they complimented each other. Mother had never had a solid-ground relationship with a man and needed someone to care for her and love her for who she was.

In time, it was obvious to everyone who knew them how special they were as a couple. Having Eddie in her life offered Mother the opportunity to expand her own horizon and to live as a free agent with no more responsibilities as the parent of a dependent child did. Mother at forty was ready for a life of her own aside from me. Eddie fulfilled this need.

Gradual Changes 4

S ome years later, I gave birth to my daughter Michele, my folks' only grandchild. With the prospect of being parents, my husband at the time, Michael Black, and I thought we could have a more productive family life out of New York City and returned to live in Minneapolis. From the time she was born, Mother and Eddie took a special interest in Michele. They loved being grandparents, doting on her and bragging about her to their friends.

Mother took time to introduce Michele to books, ideas and nature. They spent a lot of time outdoors, often taking walks around the same lakes Mother had so loved growing up.

Eddie showed Michele how to work with her hands, to repair broken items and to paint. He often took her for rides in his big Pontiac Catalina, and she enjoyed going on errands to the hardware store or the bakery with him.

Nine years later, during the summer of 1976, I choreographed a musical in St. Paul. The production required six weeks of rehearsals until the opening in September. Michele and I stayed with Mother and Eddie.

Michele found a small turtle and insisted on temporarily adopting him. Naming him Walter, she fawned over him. Walter lived with us in a makeshift fish tank on Chowen Avenue. When the show opened, it was time for Michele and me to return to our home in Washington, D.C. where we were living that year. Michele wanted to take Walter. Mother insisted on setting him free. "Walter won't like Washington, Michele. There are no lakes there," she insisted.

Michele reluctantly released him at the shore of Lake Calhoun with her grandma on hand for moral support. They both yelled, "Good bye, Walter, survive!"

Michele cried as he swam away but Mother insisted, "Look, I can see Walter doing the backstroke across the lake. He's free!"

I was always so grateful to Mother and Eddie for the care, love and time they gave Michele. The three shared a special relationship and the rapport between them was reminiscent of the bond I had with my mother all my life and with Eddie in later years. I have always felt that Mother's support and rapport with young people was one of her most endearing and enduring gifts. Eddie was unconditional love in action. Michele inherited a treasure of values from my folks.

Their marriage lasted for seventeen years. Eddie succumbed to cancer on November 26, 1978. It was a great loss to us and his passage marked the end of a special era. I remember a revealing conversation Mother and I had during the week following Eddie's death. We were sitting in her living room one evening and she looked up at me sadly, shaking her head.

"You know what is so hard about all this?" She had moved closer to me now and took my hand in hers.

"What, Mom?"

She sighed heavily as the tears began to fall and in a small, tight voice replied, "I don't have anyone to take care of anymore."

I was surprised by her candor at the time but in retrospect, I realize she was lost and didn't know what to do. Mother did continue to work a few more years. When she retired in 1984, she seemed unable to find her niche.

After Eddie's death, Mother continued to live in their house on Chowen Avenue. In 1965, she and Eddie had purchased the small, two-bedroom house with a finished basement, spacious attic, two fireplaces, and a separate two-car garage at the back, adjacent to the alley. She loved living in her own home. Mother was fierce about her privacy and loved to come home to her own space. She and Eddie had entertained frequently over the years, and enjoyed the spacious backyard just off the porch next to their bedroom.

In all the years they had occupied it, Eddie had done the yard work and general maintenance. Mother managed to keep the house in order for a while, but on her own the upkeep was beginning to overwhelm her.

Two years earlier, she had new siding put on the house, a project that took months and left her annoyed and anxious. She had hired a friend, and he put her project somewhere close to the bottom on his list of priorities.

She was frustrated and tried to call the project off, but it was already too late. The job was well underway, but subject to his availability and whim. She became noticeably agitated. When the job was finally complete she was less one friend. The home improvement episode left her angry and feeling betrayed.

I could tell Mother was looking for a change. She was restless and cross, and it was becoming evident she needed to do something about her living arrangement. It was time to leave the house with all of its old memories.

Those years spent with Eddie were precious but they were gone forever. She missed him and their life together more than she ever let on. At one point she had half-heartedly called on a local realtor for help. Even this action on her part was dragged out for months. Her actions seemed to show she wasn't as committed to selling as she pretended. She was in a rut and couldn't get enough energy to make this traumatic but necessary change.

Then something unique occurred. I was heading to a seminar one morning when a tire blew on my Volkswagen Rabbit. There I was on the side of the highway during rush hour, hoping someone would offer assistance.

A car slowed down and as it came to a stop, the driver leaned across the front seat and said, "Miss, do you need help?"

The relief I felt was obvious as I smiled back, "Oh yes, please! Could you drive me to a phone somewhere?"

He nodded and assured me saying, "We're not far from my office. It's about a half a mile from here. You can call for a tow from there."

He looked familiar. When he presented his business card, I made the connection as I recognized his name.

"Didn't you play football at one time? Are you the Ed Sharockman, who played for ten years with the Minnesota Vikings?" He nodded. During the drive to his office I learned that Ed became a real estate agent following retirement from his football career.

When we got to his office, I phoned my service station in St. Louis Park and Ed drove me back to my car, saying "I can wait with you until the tow truck comes, if you like." It was obvious that he was concerned for my safety as well as getting my car towed.

"It is kind of you to offer, but I'll be fine, really! Thanks for your help, Ed, I appreciate it."

"Well, all right. You have a good day, ok?" I opened the passenger door and got out, waving to him as he pulled out on the highway and disappeared into the stream of cars filling both lanes.

Within a few minutes, the truck arrived and towed my car into the station. My usual mechanic fixed my tire, and before long, I was on my way.

As I drove I pondered the events of the early morning and the serendipity of my rescue by a former pro football player who was now a realtor.

Later, after I shared my experience with Mother, she decided to call Mr. Sharockman about selling her house. When Mother met him, she felt completely comfortable as he instilled in her the confidence that her house would sell easily and that he was more than happy to assist her in the process.

The house on Chowen Avenue sold in nine days. For Mother, the thought of moving into the small confines of an apartment was odd, after living in a house for a total of twenty-eight years, seventeen with Eddie and eleven on her own. She selected a two-bedroom lower level flat not too far from her old residence. She wanted to stay in the neighborhood, near her lakes and the familiar places to shop. She moved the end of September of 1989.

I remember taking a day off to assist Mother in getting settled. I arrived with hammer and hooks and an upbeat attitude, hoping that she was feeling upbeat too. This change was not easy for her, but she appeared cheerful and hopeful about her new surroundings.

I put up all her pictures, and as she opened each carton, she squealed with delight over forgotten personal treasures that had been stored for years in boxes. I could see her trying to accept the change. Privately, I was hoping that her enthusiasm would continue and that she could comfortably make the transition.

For a while the change in her environment worked wonders. She seemed content with the novelty of her new surroundings. But as the weeks wore on, I noticed that every time I stopped in to see her at her new address she would find some excuse to go out. She simply did not want to spend time in her own place.

She became sullen and expressed regret about her decision to leave her old house. She found the stark white walls of her unit oppressive, and she became claustrophobic and complained of the confinement of the new space. Mother had had a problem with small spaces beginning in her youth, and this condition was starting to rear its ugly head again. She expressed the need to get out of her apartment with such frequency, I was beginning to suspect she was suffering from depression.

"I feel trapped," she would announce and then add, "I hate it here." Her agitation became more vocal and more obvious.

Mother had once told me of an experience she had when she was a young girl. An elderly neighbor had asked for Mother's help, requiring her to stay overnight. Apparently the woman's regular caregiver was unavailable, so she needed someone to substitute.

The lady was a good friend of my grandma and Mother was told she must help.

When it was time to retire for the night, the woman insisted Mother stay in the room with her and locked the door. Mother felt trapped and anxious caring for a woman in ill health. The lady was demanding and very unpleasant and when the incident was over Mother was shaken. The experience caused her to become claustrophobic.

Mother never conquered this phobia. I discovered this when I once took her through a car wash. "Chris, we're going in here?"

I thought she was joking and added with a whimsical air, "Don't worry, you're not going to drown. We're sealed in here!" She squirmed the entire time the car was being washed and settled down only when the door opened at the end of the cycle, allowing us to leave.

Mother's growing anxiety and irritability were so uncharacteristic of the woman I knew as my mother, I look back in amazement that I didn't see all the red flags in place at once when these changes began happening with regularity. It would be two years later before the mystery was solved. Hindsight is often a bitter pill we swallow when the obvious comes to the fore.

Hints and Puzzles   5

I wonder when it began exactly. Something was different, something strange, something unfamiliar, something only slightly detectable, yet present and unsettling was happening to my mother—but what?

For over a year I observed a stranger emerging from Mother. This effervescent, independent, and intelligent woman was showing some serious wear around the edges.

Had it come with her sixty-ninth birthday in June of 1987? After all, she had declared, "I'm not celebrating another one of these!"

Perhaps it was the sale of her house in the fall of 1989, a home she had lived in and lovingly taken care of for over twenty-eight years but could no longer manage.

Was it the subsequent move into an unfamiliar apartment complex that had left her moody and agitated?

There was her gradual and noticeable odd behavior too and her withdrawal from her usual daily activities. Aging didn't enter my mind. Mother was ageless in spirit.

In the spring of 1984, my free-spirited mother had recently retired and appeared to be enjoying her new lifestyle. She no longer had to adhere to a boss's demands, live by the structure of a business day, or take care of anyone except herself.

She was comfortable financially, had friends and family around her, good health, and lots of interests to fill her time. She marched to her own drum and bugle corps and always had. She amazed everyone with her originality, spirit, and vitality. Who would ever expect to have any concern about her?

In her former career as a private secretary, Mother had been creative and resourceful. She changed jobs every ten years because she needed new challenges. Mother was skilled at handling each and every job she ever had in the business world and she never burned bridges. Every employer over the years gave her high praise and great recommendations when she gave notice.

With such a profile of efficiency and career adeptness, it was difficult for me to grasp that she was now having problems with her communication skills. An emerging pattern of constantly repeating herself was disquieting and irritating to me. It simply did not fit Mother's image.

She had many friends over the years. This talent to make and keep friends of all ages spilled over into her retirement years. About this time a mutual friend of ours overheard Mother complain one day that she had never had a nickname as a child. "Helen," didn't have enough letters to justify shortening it. A friend suggested "Hels" and it stuck.

As time went on Michele, my daughter, stopped referring to my mother as Grandma, insisting instead on using Hels as so many associates now did. This change delighted Mother. In fact, she preferred being addressed as Hels for the rest of her life.

Mother was always sociable, even after she retired from corporate life. She kept in touch with her friends who were still working, and often joined them for lunch or activities following their workday. She not only continued attending gatherings of friends her own age, but was always included in parties thrown by my friends. She was welcome because she added merriment to any proceedings, usually ending up by holding court and regaling other guests with her humor and witty anecdotes. She brightened any gathering, and activity in the room focused on her. She was jovial and welcoming and loved the attention.

Comfortable in every setting, Mother would let loose by telling one of her colorful stories. She was not above patting or pinching an attractive man's derriere even if he was a stranger to her. On more than one occasion you would hear, "Hey guys, when Hels hits the room, you better back into a corner!" People loved her spontaneity and mischief.

Calling to make a date to get together with Mother was futile. She was never in and abhorred the suggestion of owning an answering machine. Her retort to my questioning her whereabouts was simply, "I've been out and about!" She was in control of her life and didn't appreciate my checking up on her.

She enjoyed being on the go. She loved to shop, dine out and take long walks. She often asked me to accompany her and we thoroughly enjoyed each other's company. The bond we shared from the time I was born continued because of the nature of our early life together: an only parent and an only child.

During these early retirement years, Mother owned an old Schwinn bicycle. Her idea of a great time was to hop on her bike and peddle down to Calhoun, Harriet and Isles, lakes connected by paths divided for pedestrians and wheel traffic.

One could begin at the first lake and cover all three in a ten-mile ride. As her momentum and stamina increased, she would peddle faster and harder until she had completed the circuit. Having given up cigarettes a decade before, Mother had developed the lung capacity of a teenager.

She never passed on the opportunity to attend a movie that always included the purchase of a giant box of popcorn. "Heavy on the butter, please," she'd emphasize.

She also still enjoyed live theatre, especially touring shows, preferably musicals.

At home, reading was a favorite activity. She chose novels written by Lawrence Sanders because to her his writing was intriguing and fast-paced.

On casual outings her favorite indulgence was a double thick chocolate malt topped with whipped cream. She could polish off the entire glass and then finish the last small dollop remaining in the metal mixing container. She was a regular at Bridgeman's, the local ice cream store, as she often expressed the need for "something chocolate or butterscotch."

A year after her retirement in 1985, she had joined a health club and become religious about her attendance, swimming at least six times a week. She swam laps and because of her incredible endurance, swam at least a mile each visit. Enthralled with this activity, she eagerly looked forward to mornings at the pool. She believed a large pool should be used for lap swimming and reserved for serious swimmers. She guarded her lap lane with ferocity until she had completed her regimen, having no patience with individuals loafing around the pool or people engaged in water aerobics. Entering the pool she felt instant joy and once remarked, "When I am immersed in that water doing my laps, a certain peace comes over me." For Mother, a daily swim was her meditation.

One time she told me about an incident that had occurred on one of her regular workout days.

"Chrissy, I went into the locker room to get ready for my morning swim. I walked out into the pool area and suddenly noticed a man standing mid-pool just gaping at me. Well, I knew my figure was pretty good but not that good. I looked around and there was no one else in the area. I couldn't figure out what he was looking at until I looked down. I was naked. I was standing there holding my swimming suit in my hand. I couldn't believe it! I was so embarrassed that I just gave up, got dressed and went home." Though I was surprised hearing the story, I wasn't concerned by Mother's *faux pas*. It did create quite a funny picture. Later when I retold the story to a close friend, he laughed too.

"That sounds like something Hels would do!"

"Doesn't it?"

"It's so typical of her."

"That's my mother!"

We both agreed it was a great story and then I let it go, thinking no more about it.

On another occasion, again at the club, Mother apparently forgot to lock her locker when she left the changing area. After her swim, she showered, dressed and realized that her purse was missing. In a panic, she reported the missing purse at the front desk. Her car and house keys were in the purse and she was forced to leave her car parked at the club. A staff person volunteered to drive her to her apartment. Once home, she had someone from the management office let her in with a master key. Worst of all, her wallet, her credit cards and checkbook were all in the purse. She called and reported the theft to her bank. Later, a neighbor drove her back to the club to retrieve her car. Mother was shaken by the experience and mentioned it several times that week.

Being as gregarious as Mother had always been, it was puzzling to notice that she was leaving her apartment less and less. This was not her style. A few years later, I was gradually aware that she was becoming depressed and withdrawn. She napped frequently during the day and would not bother to answer the phone. This concerned me because Mother and I had always spoken to each other daily, and because she was becoming reclusive of late I took the initiative to suggest activities. When I succeeded in getting her to go out she wasn't very adventuresome, wanting to do the same things over and over. Going to the movies or out to eat were becoming her main interest.

Mother was also beginning to show an intense attraction to men. She started dating men years younger than herself. I noticed she came on strong to strangers and most of her conversations contained innuendoes.

This development of indiscriminate, overbearing and flirtatious behavior toward men was unflattering at her age. She had always flirted with select individuals but now she was coming on to every man she encountered. On one occasion she phoned me at the office to ask if a friend of mine could bring her a tax form on his lunch hour. He worked near the post office and her apartment. Mother asked about him frequently so this particular request was no surprise, but I knew he would be uncomfortable, so I stopped by the post office and picked up the form for her. She never mentioned my friend again.

As I became more consciously observant, I began to notice Mother's escalating anxiety and irritability. She was becoming possessive too. On one occasion I mentioned to her that my good friends Joel Thom and Wayne Harrington had asked me to join them at a lake retreat to celebrate my birthday in a few weeks.

"Mom, it's a wonderful opportunity to have a vacation from the city and relax for a few days, and you know how much fun they are to be around," I enthused.

I knew she enjoyed their company as well and was surprised when she objected, "I'd prefer you stayed in town. I want you to celebrate your birthday with me. Why do you have to go up to some lake, anyway?"

I was quite surprised by her testy response and disappointed by her resistance and selfish attitude. However, I decided to stay in town, not wishing to hurt her feelings when the date arrived. We simply went out to dinner, something that was not that special and could have been scheduled a day or two ahead or after my invitation to visit the lake with my friends.

A dear friend of Mother's bought a new car and drove it over to show her. When she left, I could tell that Mother was irritated. "I don't know why she deserves a new car. I'm the one who needs one," she commented.

I stopped in my tracks, not believing what I had just heard. She continued a barrage of slights toward her old friend. "She's just showing off. I can't stand her. She has a lot of nerve!"

I finally said, "It isn't very becoming of you to act like this."

She barked back, "I don't give a damn if you think it's unbecoming!" I retreated from the exchange a bit shaken and said nothing more.

During this time I discovered that Mother wasn't eating a balanced diet. Her refrigerator contained only an orange or two, some Perrier water, a container of yogurt and a few slices of bread. Her cupboard held a few cans of beans and little else. On her own at home she apparently wasn't eating much. However, she liked to go to The Great Wall, a Chinese restaurant in the neighborhood, and when I took her out for a meal she ate well, her appetite apparently strong. And when the meal was over, she began insisting on dessert. In fact, her yen for sweets was growing at a surprising rate.

Another change that troubled me was Mother's lack of interest in traveling to Hawaii to spend a few weeks of the winter with her brother Paul and his family. For the past five consecutive winters she had visited them and stayed for at least a month. When I offered to go to her travel agent with her to arrange the trip, she found first one excuse and then another to put it off. This change of heart was a departure from her usual enthusiasm for escaping a winter in Minnesota.

My awareness of changes in Mother continued to crystallize on her birthday June 7th, that puzzling year 1991. Mother had always celebrated birthdays with enthusiasm, especially her own. Arranging to take the afternoon off from my job in order to take her to lunch, I arrived at her apartment with colorful presents that she opened with relish. She loved clothes and I had carefully selected summer clothes in all the colors she loved. Among her gifts was a special surprise: a red satin, floor length robe styled to fit Joan Crawford.

"Oh, Chrissy, I saw Joan in one just like this in *Mildred Pierce*. It's just fabulous! I have to try it on, now!"

Mother squealed as she put her arm in each sleeve slipping on the robe and tying the sash around her waist. Flouncing around the living room, she vamped an imaginary swain, enticing him into her boudoir.

She continued to open the remaining gifts, a set of orange sweats and yellow shorts with a matching top. She giggled in anticipation of each wrapped treasure, and as she opened each package she held up her new outfit for show. Mother was easy to shop for because she wore clothes well and appreciated everything she received.

Since it was getting late, and not wanting us to lose our lunch reservation, I suggested we put all her new gifts in her bedroom closet on a shelf high out of Chessie's reach. Chessie was her beautiful Maine Coon cat with a magnificent long, shining coat and voluminous tail that she waved in regal fashion. She was a grand animal and she knew it, but she was also a mischievous rascal.

We left for lunch. I had selected Ikebana, a new Japanese restaurant in the fashionable Warehouse District in downtown Minneapolis. A client had recommended it highly. During lunch our conversation covered all the usual ground, and we thoroughly enjoyed our meal. After lunch, I suggested we stop by to see her nephew Greg Winter. He and his wife Nancy were hosting a bridal shower the next day for his sister Lucinda who was getting married in a few weeks. She and Mother had developed a close bond when she lived with Mother for a few months following college. Mother was pleased Lucinda was getting married, and she was delighted with her niece's choice, Jim Ankeny, an affable and talented young fellow.

When we arrived at Greg's house, Mother's brother Vernon and his wife Cecilia were also there, having just arrived from Michigan. Everyone was busy helping with the shower details. The group was chatting as we walked into the kitchen, and there was an air of excitement among the family.

I greeted everyone enthusiastically but Mother remained silent. Her silence soon became obvious to everyone because she usually took over a room. The chatting gradually stopped, and another minute of awkward silence went by before Vernon said, "Hi, Sis, how are you?"

Mother stared blankly at her brother.

Greg approached his aunt with his usual bear hug, saying, "Aunt Helen, good to see you!" Mother continued to look confused and did not respond to his greeting.

In my usual fashion, I made up the silence with repartee. "It's good to see you Uncle Vern." I reached out to hug him in my usual way.

"It's nice to see you, Christine."

Then, I reached out for his wife. "Cecilia, it's been a long time."

"How have you been dear?"

"Just great!" I then looked at the kitchen area that had been enlarged and commented, "Nancy, the house looks so beautiful. I can't wait for the shower tomorrow. Is there anything we can bring?"

Nancy responded warmly saying, "Just bring yourselves!"

Trying all the while to cover up Mother's obvious unresponsiveness, I realized she had no idea where she was though she had been to Greg and Nancy's home many times over the years. Conversation began again and continued to swirl around the room but Mother didn't contribute one comment to the familiar family topics. She stood silently by my side. As the strain was building in the room, I suggested that we leave. Saying goodbye to everyone, I led Mother out of the kitchen, through the side door and down the long driveway to the car.

Mother's strange behavior left me feeling a little shaky but I feigned nonchalance. On the way home I stopped at a store to buy a shower card for Lucinda.

"Who is the card for?" Mother was clearly confused.

"I am buying a card to go with my shower gift for Lucinda."

"Why are you giving her a shower gift?"

"Mom, Lucinda is getting married in a few weeks. Don't you remember?"

Apparently she hadn't remembered a thing about the upcoming wedding or that I had helped her pick out a shower gift recently.

I couldn't figure out what was going on. It didn't make sense. I was growing impatient and a bit bewildered myself, but I kept the lid on myself as we drove back to her apartment. I was shaken by Mother's behavior at Greg's house. It was now around five in the afternoon.

When we entered the apartment, I decided to change the subject of weddings and distracted Mother by mentioning the new clothes. We went into the bedroom, and I reached up into the closet and lifted the gifts down. She watched as I spread the clothing out on the bed, pointing out each colorful outfit.

Mother looked surprised. "Where did these come from?"

"What do you mean, Mom?"

"This clothing!" She picked up the red satin robe as though for the first time. "And this yellow outfit?"

"These are your birthday presents that you opened earlier this afternoon."

She looked puzzled as though I was playing a game with her. "These are from you?"

"Yes. Don't you remember? I gave them to you before we went to lunch." She couldn't remember. She only looked blank but then added, "Thanks." Nothing I said seemed to register. It was as though she couldn't remember it was her birthday. Now I was feeling more than uneasy. I was frightened.

For the first time, the odd, previously disconnected incidents began to take on a shape. Instead of being just puzzled, I became deeply concerned.

The whole experience at Greg's house was alarming. I didn't want to upset Mother by allowing my growing fear to register on my face. Mother's behavior was extremely unsettling.

The time had come to step back and assess the situation. Would something have to be done? What? I couldn't live in this limbo created by her uncharacteristic behavior that had been going on for months. I went home resolved to approach Mother with my concerns. When I did, a drama began from which there was no turning back.

Alarm and Questions   6

M y mind reeled as I thought of ways to approach Mother. This was not going to be easy. I had never interfered in her business before. She was my mother, and I was her kid. She was a very independent person and I respected her privacy.

Now it appeared I had to interfere. I had no idea what was happening to Mother except that I was convinced she might be in some kind of trouble. As proud as she was, she would never admit it.

I was going to have to take a stand and use a good old movie line like "The jig is up." I was nervous at the thought of such a conversation, a confrontation with my own mother.

When I could stand this feeling of uncertainty no longer, I made the call that I had dreaded. "Hi, Mom. Do you feel like going out for some breakfast?"

"I think that would be lovely."

"Good! I'll pick you up at nine sharp, ok?"

"Sounds like a plan. See you then."

I got into the shower. As the soothing spray of warm water cascaded over me, I thought back to a time when everything about life had seemed normal. Mother was enjoying her retirement and going about her business, a free-spirited lady with time to fill as it pleased her. I thought how carefree she was.

In my mind, the picture of her wheeling around the lakes, swimming laps and walking briskly around the nature walk behind her apartment complex brought me to tears. I had a large, heavy spot of sadness in the center of my chest. Things were changing and would be different forever. There I stood in the shower, water and tears running down my face.

It was a warm June morning, and I had the windows down on my old blue Rabbit as I drove to pick up Mother and take her to breakfast. My feeling on the drive to the McDonald's across from my former high school in St. Louis Park can best be described as tense. Sitting across from each other at the table, we made small talk and joked and chatted, munching on Egg McMuffins. She sipped black coffee and I had my usual, tea with milk.

We finished our food, and I turned to her and looked her in the eyes. I remember thinking the whole world around me had been scrubbed away and it was just the two of us. Our little table was floating in the stratosphere and we were the only people in the Universe. The time had come.

"Mom, I have to tell you that I have noticed some changes."

"Oh?" She sipped her coffee, crushing the wrapper her breakfast had come in.

My mouth was dry and my hands were shaking. She just sat quietly and took in every word. "Mom, something is wrong and I have to get you to a doctor!"

I was stumbling over the words as I spoke. "There, I actually said it," I thought to myself. I waited for a response.

Mother stared back at me for a moment and then she looked down at the table. Tears ran down her face.

"Oh thank God, you care!" She knew. All this time she had been suspended in some incomprehensible void, knowing something was happening to her.

I stammered back, "Well of course I care. I love you. Things have not been right for sometime. Don't worry, we will get you a complete work-up!"

"Ok." She began to calm down as my heart rate accelerated. She sat there, staring ahead and then she leaned on her forearms and began trembling.

I moved over and sat next to her. Putting my arms around her, I tried comforting her. "Don't worry, Mom. Everything is going to be all right."

Though my attitude and voice had the bravado of a take-charge individual, my stomach was fluttering with nerves. I smiled to myself thinking of a remark made years earlier by my former acting teacher. He was giving an example of overcoming stage fright saying, "Though you have butterflies in your stomach, tell them to fly in formation!"

We left McDonald's and I drove Mother home. We were silent. Familiar blocks of familiar houses slipped past unnoticed.

When I pulled up in front of her building she took my hand for a moment, squeezed it, and said calmly, "Thank you, dear, for your concern." She got out of the car, walked to the front door and turned to wave as I pulled away from the curb. I kept thinking, as I backed up and watched her enter her building and disappeared from view, that I could never love her more than I did at that moment.

The next Monday, I called Mother's clinic, Park-Nicollet in St. Louis Park. A brisk voice at the other end of the line recited, "Please call the department of Senior Concerns." I dialed and heard another brisk voice say, "This is the department of Senior Concerns. How may I help you?"

"I would like to make an appointment for my mother, Helen LaCaze." I was abruptly put on hold. I was agitated. After what seemed like an enormous wait, the receptionist returned.

"The next available appointment is in two months."

"Two months! You have nothing available sooner?" My voice was rising in a frustrated and shrill crescendo. Two months seemed like an endless amount of time to wait. Two months to wait to unravel this developing, knotted puzzle; two months to wait to solve a mystery. I made the August appointment for her and in doing so felt a wave of relief rush over me. The doctors would take care of it.

I considered the toll age might be taking on Mother. Was she really getting old? I was not ready for her to be old. In my mind, I was standing on the edge of a cliff. At any moment a big gust of wind would blow me from the edge and I would fall to the bottom of the chasm below.

In the meantime, we discussed going to a special event, like a play or touring production and Mother insisted on treating, saying, "I'll take care of it, Chris." The subject never came up again. Later, I found cash, a large amount of cash in a drawer that she had set aside to purchase the tickets. When I asked her about the money I had found, she giggled and said, "It's for something or other. I don't remember."

I was going to turn fifty that summer. Mother had always loved celebrating my birthday and had made a point of spending that time with me, but as the day grew closer that year she never mentioned it.

I thought that fifty was a milestone number for a birthday. My friends Joel Thom and Wayne Harrington thought so too. They planned a reception commemorating my day and invited a large group of associates and friends to their home in my honor. Mother attended but appeared to be confused about the reason for the celebration. She was drinking during the gathering and was having trouble putting her words together in intelligible sentences.

Two former acting students of mine, acquainted with Mother for a number of years, took me aside. "What's wrong with Hels? She's out of it and stumbling around in the back yard."

"What do you mean?" I pulled together a cool posture, feigning nonchalance at the remark.

"She doesn't seem herself."

"Oh, she's probably had a cocktail or two," I remarked lamely. When I could break away from our huddle, I found my daughter Michele. "Try to steer Hels away from the bar, ok?"

Michele understood immediately and went to find her grandma.

The party continued but I remained preoccupied by the earlier remark, "She doesn't seem herself." The event should have been a celebration for me, but instead I felt an undercurrent of sadness. I was worried about Mother's increasing inability to recognize people. And drinking wasn't helping her. She didn't seem able to handle liquor anymore. It added to her confusion and made her look like a drunk instead of the witty woman she had always been. Was she becoming an alcoholic?

Following the party, she was exhausted and wanted to go to bed. I took her home and after making sure she was tucked in, left her apartment emotionally and physically drained. I was only too happy to return home and fall into a stress-free sleep.

Days later, Mother and I decided to take in a movie and have dinner. It was the end of July and the Minnesota weather was beautiful. We agreed that she would drive over to my place and we would go from there. I waited. Time ticked away and there was no sign of her. I watched out the window for her red Ford. An hour passed. I finally dialed her number. She answered immediately with an agitated, barely audible voice.

It was hard to keep the impatience out of my voice. "When are you coming over? I thought we had plans!"

After a long pause she said, "Chris, I can't remember how to get to your house."

"What do you mean?" I could not fathom what she was talking about.

"Please give me directions, dear."

"You've driven the route for years. How can you not remember?"

I couldn't believe she was having difficulty remembering such an easy drive. Irritated, I recited directions as though I was a drill sergeant talking to a new recruit and hung up.

After a few minutes, during which I consciously tried to calm down, I spotted Mother pulling up to the house. She was having trouble parking the car, pulling forward and backing in several times. I went downstairs and walked to the curb. As she got out of the car, I hugged her and calmly told her we would have to go to a different showing of the film because we were late. She nodded and we climbed into my car. She insisted that I drive. After her initial confusion, we followed our plan to attend a movie and get a bite to eat afterward. We had a wonderful time, which dispelled my earlier irritation with her.

Lucinda and Jim's wedding day arrived in early August. Mother and I attended the ceremony and later the reception. It was a delightful day. Remembering her behavior at my birthday party, I insisted that Mother have only soft drinks during the party. She didn't question my request. However her confusion was obvious. She failed to recognize a number of the guests in attendance, many of whom were friends and relatives.

"Chrissy, who is that?" Mother was pointing to an attractive brunette who I recognized as a close friend of Lucinda's.

"That's Claire, Mom."

"Who's Claire?"

"Mom, Claire is one of Lucinda's best friends. She came with Lucinda to visit you many times on Chowen."

"Oh."

Mother spotted another young woman who looked familiar, but again she couldn't make the connection. "Chrissy, who is that?"

"Mom, that's Sheila. She's Lucinda's other best friend."

There was no response or acknowledgment, so I changed the subject and we continued to mingle.

Mother didn't respond to others she had been on friendly terms with before. I heard whispers among our relatives. They appeared to notice that she was not her usual, direct self.

Lucinda's oldest brother Jeff was visibly puzzled when he asked his aunt Helen to join him on the dance floor and she declined. Aunt Helen refusing to dance?

Others noticed how passive she was, sitting to one side, staring at the activity, not participating. She didn't remember names, seemed distant even with her closest relatives including her brother Vernon and wouldn't speak unless prompted. I was relieved when the reception was over and I could take her home.

Social gatherings were becoming a strange challenge for her. Could she really be getting that old so suddenly?

A short time later, Lucinda mentioned to me that she wondered if there was something wrong. Aunt Helen hadn't seemed herself at the wedding.

She said her first hint that something was different occurred on the day when Mother and I had stopped by to assist her with her wedding invitations.

"Do you remember when Helen was putting stamps on the reply envelopes?"

"Vaguely."

"Well, she kept putting the stamps on the opposite corner of the envelope from where the stamps are required to be placed for mailing."

"You know, come to think of it, you're right! I do remember something strange about that."

"Well, I didn't want to draw attention to her or embarrass her in any way."

"I seem to remember you gave her another assignment…sealing the envelopes, wasn't it?"

"Yes."

That incident had occurred in the early summer of 1991 before I could recognize Mother's problems.

Mother's mystery impairment appeared sporadically. One day she was lucid and conversational, and the next, vague and nervous. There was no consistency to her behavior. The bottom line was I had to guide her with patience. Evidence of the changes in her behavior was not waning; it was mounting.

On one occasion I spotted Mother coming out of the building across from her own. She was heading to her car parked in front of the building she had just exited.

"Hi, Mom, where are you going?"

"I'm going home."

"Mom, you are home!"

"Ok, Chris."

She then proceeded to take her car key and open the door of her car. As she bent down to get into her vehicle, I physically cringed at her obvious confusion. She was not more than thirty feet from her front door.

Trying to stay calm, I walked over and gently took hold of her hand. I led Mother across the parking area to her building and to her apartment. Once inside I eased the keys out of her hand. I shook my head in troubled amazement as I returned to my car.

Mother had always been an infallible organizer, largely from developing the skill as an executive secretary. She was adept at keeping excellent and accurate records and this carried over to handling her personal finances. She was always savvy with money.

Now in the late summer of 1991, Mother missed a rent payment for the first time in her life. She was upset when she received a reminder notice from the front office of her complex.

I asked to see her checkbook, something I had never done before. As I looked through her check register, it was obvious that she had forgotten the rent was due on the first of the month. Pointing this out as diplomatically as I could, she remarked, "Oh no, I forgot!"

We sat down and with my help, she painstakingly made out a check and I took it over to the office immediately. This omission was clearly a sign of trouble ahead.

Anticipation 7

I felt relief and dread all at the same time as I drove Mother to her appointment at the clinic. Our two months of waiting had passed.

We sat down in the reception area, waiting to be called. I was attempting to make small talk as my eyes darted about the room. Mother was in good spirits. I thought if I just talked a lot, it would distract us both.

What seemed like an eternity passed before the attending nurse called Mother's name. Ellie Bisek had the smile of an angel and the gusto of Mrs. Santa Claus. She was direct yet kind and nurturing.

Ellie reminded me of my first favorite teacher, when I was a little kid. She led us down a long corridor to a large examination room where she began the interview by asking the usual questions.

I could see her bonding with my mother. Mother relaxed and began enjoying herself and I began to relax as well. After months of struggle and guesswork I felt she was safe in capable hands. After all, doctors with their modern medicine can identify and cure almost anything. Whatever was wrong, they would take care of it. Dr. Sharon Marx, the attending physician, was a specialist in gerontology.

When I was able to get Dr. Marx alone from deep inside me came the question, "Could my mother's difficulty be from Alzheimer's?" The notion that what was wrong with Mother was more than just old age had occurred to me a few weeks previously. I had done some thinking about other possibilities. I felt if I could put a name on whatever was wrong, a doctor would be able to treat and cure it.

Just where that strange word "Alzheimer's" came from, I didn't know. Maybe I had heard it on a made-for-television movie. I had picked up a book on the subject at a neighborhood bookstore and had skimmed through it. The word itself sounded sinister to me. It seemed mysterious, perverse, and ugly.

Trying to throw a little reassurance my way, Dr. Marx replied, "We don't like to assume that it's Alzheimer's immediately."

As she explained the diagnostic tests that Mother would undergo, I realized there was no direct answer at the moment.

The doctor explained that they look for the cause of behavioral changes by the process of elimination first. They test for metabolic disturbances in the body, initiate cognitive testing, brain scans and all the other means to find conclusive proof that some other disease is developing.

I asked, "Is there absolute proof of the disease's presence or is it mostly assumption based on the tests conducted? Or do you recognize the disease process unfolding through stages of deterioration?" I learned that a prior arrangement could be made to prove that the individual died from complications due to Alzheimer's. I could sign an agreement stating that an autopsy be performed after Mother passed away. This procedure, I was told, is the only means of proving conclusively that Alzheimer's was present.

During the autopsy, the examiner finds the neurofibullar tangles in the brain tissue, as well as secretions of plaque created by the over-production of beta-amyloid fluid that attaches to the neurons like sludge in the brain folds. This finding is concrete evidence of the disease.

That was too much information all at once. I was not prepared to deal with that kind of decision at the moment.

As September passed, Mother submitted to a series of appointments that included a physical and lab work-up, an MRI, basic problem-solving, psychological testing and therapy sessions.

Ellie proved to be a comforting friend. She was aware of Mother's need for support, and her compassion extended to our immediate family while we waited for the results.

Ellie called me in mid-September. "Chris, based on my observation of your mother and the results of her testing, I think we can safely say that she is in the early stages of Alzheimer's."

"Oh God! What does that mean? What do we do now?"

"First, do you need to tell her?"

"Yes, out of respect for my mother."

"When do you want to do it?"

"When is a good time to tell anyone that?" My eyes were welling up and I couldn't catch my breath.

Now "something" had a name: Alzheimer's. That seemed better but didn't help as much as I thought it would.

I knew from my reading that the disease was incurable and fatal. Mother was going to deteriorate gradually, and we were going to have to watch it.

"I'd like to tell her as soon as possible. My mother is an intelligent and truthful person. I want to be truthful with her."

"How about at her therapy session next week?"

"Yes, the sooner the better. Thanks."

With my stomach in knots, I remembered Mother's eerie remark a year earlier, "Chris, I could stand to lose anything except my mind." Ironically, she had jokingly referred to her repetitious conversations by saying, "It must be my Alzheimer's!"

Today, I found little humor in the remark. Her comment tossed off at the time, became a chilling prophecy. It seemed as if the truth really was stranger than fiction.

The day came to tell Mother. I made the appointment to meet with Ellie and Dr. Marx. Michele joined us. As we assembled, I looked over at Mother and the expression on her face told me everything. She looked defeated. If she had been waving a white flag, it wouldn't have been more obvious. Michele and I furtively glanced at one another. Mother looked small and vulnerable. The verdict came from Ellie.

"Hels, you are in the early stages of Alzheimer's Disease. What do you think about this?"

"I feel like going out and getting loaded, but I know it won't do any good."

Mother hadn't missed a beat. She had responded in her true fashion, with honesty and humor.

Mother never again remarked about her diagnosis following the meeting.

Before we left, I took Ellie aside.

"Where do we go from here?"

"I will continue to see Hels for therapy for awhile, and I think it would be helpful for you and Michele to sit in during the sessions in case you have any questions, ok?"

"Ok, Ellie. You've been so kind to my mother and to us. Thank you."

I needed all the help I could get at this point. She put her hand on my sleeve and gave me a weak smile. I turned to Michele who gave me a look that seemed to say, "Let's get out of here!"

We left the clinic and drove Mother home. On the ride back to her apartment, she chatted with Michele as though she either rejected or refused to believe the news, or perhaps she had forgotten it. Either way, it was hard to read her thoughts. She could be in denial, or perhaps she did what she had always done, pulled herself up by the bootstraps and went on. No matter what Mother may have been thinking after our meeting with the doctor, she never showed resentment.

In the weeks that followed, I dispensed medication to Mother, prescribed for depression. A by-product of the disease in the early stage is depression. Because Mother had such trouble remembering, I couldn't rely on her to take the medication, so I stopped over every day to make sure she took it. I thought to myself, "Who wouldn't be depressed about being told you had Alzheimer's Disease? Imagine knowing you have the disease as it robs you of your communication skills, functioning, personality, and saddest of all, your memories."

One evening, some weeks after our meeting with the doctor, I was getting ready to go home after having spent a few hours with Mother. I was putting on my jacket in the front hallway, when I looked over at her and saw her staring at me.

Her eyes held a terror that was frightening. She crossed the room and hugged me with all of her strength. Her arms were trembling as she spoke in a voice that sounded distorted and thin. "Chris, I'm so scared, don't leave me!"

I held on to her with an equally tight grip and tried to speak to her softly. "Mom, you raised me and you've always had my best interest at heart. Don't you think it is my turn now?" Her arms relaxed as she tried to smile through her panic.

"Oh Chris, I love you!"

"I love you too, Mom."

We stood together for a time and cried.

Looking back, it is clear to me now that several odd incidents occurred what must have been the beginning of her development of Alzheimer's. Each time I had found it amusing or strange but had pushed the thought away, thinking it was characteristic of her personality. I loved her eccentric and unique character and her lack of concern about what people thought of her. She had always let everything roll off her back until now.

After that evening, I settled in and readied myself for what I'd come to think of as "the journey." We would begin and end an odyssey together. The trip would be challenging and uncertain at times. I would be facing an enemy that was merciless and unstoppable. This trip would unfold for years to come.

"That" Disease 8

T he whole thing was unthinkable, unreasonable. I felt as though I was in the middle of a nightmare and that I would soon wake up. After the initial diagnosis, I needed time to accept the prognosis for Mother in the early stages of Alzheimer's Disease. There was no turning back.

Cruelest of all was the fact that Mother was in perfect physical health at the time of her diagnosis. I could not recall a time in her life that she had been faced with a major illness or a surgical procedure. Her once-a-year cold would vanish after three days, and she only took aspirin when the first sniffles began. Her facile mind would deteriorate long before her body did.

I began trying to piece together the history of this horrendous development. Since early 1990, I had detected something strange in Mother's behavior. As I mulled over past occurrences, suddenly little details began to coalesce in my thoughts.

I thought back over the past year and a half of her often-puzzling behavior and realized that I had first noticed subtle differences in her after Eddie's death and more so after she sold her home and moved to an apartment complex. Although the new place was close to her old neighborhood, the move in September 1989 was a big change for her.

I remembered her anxiety over minor occurrences that never would have upset her before; the repetitious conversation, the missed appointments, forgetting to put on her swimming suit before entering the pool area at her club. She cleverly concealed her struggle to keep herself together. When she repeated herself over and over and it had become noticeable enough for us to comment on it, she'd laughed and said, "It must be my Alzheimer's!" Mother was always quick with a quip or remark. She never let on when she was distressed. People of her generation grew up believing that in times of trial one should put on a stiff upper lip.

I was beginning to understand that what was happening to her must have been terrifying, yet she never let on. When her thoughts would jumble or sudden gaps in her memory occurred, she would plough right through those hideous moments and act as if nothing was unusual.

After agonizing over Mother's diagnosis, I came to accept that I had no control over her fate. Her gradual decline was inevitable, and I couldn't change the course of her illness no matter how much I prayed for a different scenario. This disease named by Dr. Alois Alzheimer in 1906 was controlling her, and the only control I had was over my attitude.

The first thing I did was to read every bit of factual information I could get my hands on. I gathered statistics, talked to informed sources and to a probate attorney who was acquainted with Mother. I found useful information through the caregivers, families and professionals who were dealing with the disease.

Someone recommended I read the bible of the caregiver The Thirty-Six Hour Day. This book is a compilation of caregivers' collected experience written for the layperson. It describes the four stages of the disease and a step-by-step approach to them. It is a factual and detailed reference.

I had purchased the book just before I left on a vacation. I threw it in my suitcase, thinking I would read it while I was away. For days the book lay unopened in my bag. I couldn't bring myself to read it.

I was afraid to learn too much too soon. I didn't feel I was ready. I thought, "Ready for what?" The irony was that the answer lay in becoming better informed about the disease's progression.

Those pages contained the cold, hard facts. I felt intimidated and overwhelmed, and I hadn't even opened the book!

I was gripped by the fear of the unknown. I was alone and was facing monumental decisions concerning Mother's well-being. As her only child, the decisions I made concerning Mother's welfare would directly affect the quality of the rest of her life. I didn't realize yet that no matter what I decided, the disease would run its course in its own way.

Finally with one day remaining of vacation, I picked up the book. Glancing through the table of contents my eyes fell on the chapter subtitle dealing with love. I immediately opened to that chapter and began to read.

As I read, I learned I had a gift right inside myself that would see me through the task of guiding Mother as her illness progressed. The gift was my love for her. At that exact moment my fear lifted and I knew what I had to do. My commitment was in place.

A second word in that chapter, acceptance, had the most impact. To accept was to make peace with reality. Mother was going to deteriorate. There was no power in the Universe to change this fact. I knew the only way to care for her was with love, patience, respect and understanding.

I learned that Alzheimer's is an incurable degeneration of the brain. The disease ranks fourth as the leading cause of death following heart disease, cancer and stroke. Estimates at the time of Mother's diagnosis in September of 1991 stated the disease develops in forty-seven percent of the adult population over eighty-five years of age.

At the present time, four million Americans are afflicted. By the year 2025, unless a cure is found, it is estimated that twenty-two million people will have the disease worldwide.

Research has produced drugs that aid patients by maintaining their ability to concentrate so that they can sustain their quality of life longer. The medication is usually administered to those in the early stage of the disease. Scientists continue to focus on finding a cure.

The Alzheimer's Association became a rock I hung onto in a stormy lake, and it could get stormy caring for Mother. I could arm myself with information and realistically deal with the changes in her, knowing they were coming. I had to let go of my fear and denial in order to get through this experience.

Ready to hear it all, I joined several support groups. I found I was not alone, although in the beginning I felt singled out and set apart from the rest of the world. I attended a seminar to get information about procedures to follow. My attendance was necessary but I felt odd being there. Standing at a hospitality table writing out a name badge, I noticed a woman staring at me from across the room. She approached.

"Didn't you go to St. Louis Park High? You look so familiar!"

I studied her for a moment and remarked, "You look very familiar too."

She studied me as well and then a flicker of recognition crossed her face. "Weren't you a Parkette?"

I was suddenly back in 1957 as I made the connection. "Oh my gosh, Jane Ann Riebe!"

I had suddenly remembered that Jane Ann was an upperclassman during my sophomore year in high school. We were original members of the Parkettes, a precision kick line styled after the Radio City Rockettes, and the first in the Lake Conference to perform at basketball games during halftime.

We talked for a long time, and with each passing moment she made me aware that there was a large family of people all sharing the same situation. Her mother had the disease and had moved to a nursing home. Jane Ann faced the task of selecting the right facility for her. We were all seeing a loved one through a challenging disease that he or she couldn't get through without our help.

I sat the entire day at this seminar soaking up information like the proverbial sponge. I left the conference feeling empowered, enlightened and ready to do battle with the enemy, Alzheimer's.

Mother was having difficulty handling her own affairs. I was already monitoring her bills and finances. Living on her own, isolated and uncertain of her condition, she lived in an anxious cloud, trying to function.

I had to stay one step ahead of the enemy on this new battlefield and I needed a step-by-step game plan. Years before, Mother had met a probate lawyer, Skip Lefler, through her nephew Jeffrey Winter and had him assist her in doing a will. As their relationship grew Mother came to rely on him as a source of legal advice. I obtained his number and called him. He agreed to meet with me to discuss what I would need to do legally on behalf of Mother. We set up a meeting that week at a coffee café in the uptown area of Minneapolis.

At our first encounter that took place in the fall of 1991, shortly after Mother's diagnosis, Skip explained all the ramifications of applying for conservatorship.

"In this role through appointment by the court you will have total control over your mother's physical and financial well-being," he explained. I sat across from him hanging on every word.

"You will handle her monthly income through a direct-deposit conservator account you will open." I leaned in, trying to process all the details.

Skip continued to explain the procedure adding, "This must be arranged before your day in court." Sipping on his coffee, he wrote notes on a yellow-lined pad, glancing up occasionally as our conversation continued.

My mind was reeling, and I was beginning to develop a headache. "You mean I will make decisions about treatment and decide where she lives?

"That's correct. As your mother's conservator you will be required to attend a hearing at the end of each fiscal year, and as your attorney, I will submit her financial records."

I felt overwhelmed by all the information and Skip was aware of that. He was an excellent probate lawyer and was used to dealing with civilians. He offered to handle all the accounting. A wave of relief passed over me. He told me that it would take a few months to be scheduled on the court's calendar to expedite my appointment as conservator.

I thanked him for his time and left the restaurant with the weight of the world on my shoulders. My headache had turned to exhaustion. I was completely overwhelmed with the enormity of the task ahead, but I had gained another knowledgeable ally in Skip.

When Mother and I made tentative plans together she would ask, "Would you write it down?"

At first this request puzzled me. I was just learning about Alzheimer's, and I couldn't fully grasp that a formerly brilliant businesswoman needed assistance in remembering an appointment. As the weeks passed, I became an expert in writing notes to remind Mother of details her mind could not hold on to.

During an impressive career as an executive secretary, her dictation speed was 125 words per minute and now I watched her deciphering simple notes and lists with difficulty.

I became irritated and impatient with her fumbling, but in time I realized what was happening to her. No matter how many reminders I left her she could no longer rely on her memory. Written words had lost their meaning for her. My irritation and impatience turned into compassion.

One afternoon, I stopped by to make sure Mother was taking her anti-depressants. I knocked several times, but she didn't answer the door. Frustrated, I opened her door with the extra key I always carried.

She was gone. I looked out her front window and noticed that her red car was parked at the curb in front of her building. At least she wasn't driving. She had forgotten I was coming, in spite of the fact that I had called to remind her that I would be stopping by after work. Where could she have walked to by herself? Was she lost?

Mother was used to taking walks in beautiful weather. She loved to go out and get an ice cream cone, and as I thought about her whereabouts, I realized she was probably at the Dairy Queen a few blocks from her apartment.

Driving Excelsior Boulevard, the main drag near her complex, I spotted her sitting on a bench in the parking lot of the Dairy Queen. Sitting next to her was a sizeable woman with a wonderful smile and a cheery demeanor. Joyce Fowler, I discovered through our conversation, lived in the building next door to Mother. She had invited Joyce to join her for an ice cream cone and together they had walked the few blocks to the store.

Joyce and Mother liked each other, and they became friends. She was kind and often came around to check on Mother or keep her company. Joyce offered to cook meals occasionally, and would watch television with Mother in the evenings. She was good at distracting her and filling the gap when she needed companionship. Joyce had no idea my mother was struggling with Alzheimer's. When I took her aside and explained her disease, Joyce was shocked.

"I don't understand, Chrissy, your mom seems so with it!" I smiled a knowing smile in response to Joyce's remark.

"She covers well."

"You mean she's faking it?"

"This is her way of coping and trying to control her world." Joyce seemed to understand and because she was a compassionate person, she continued to keep Mother company whenever she could.

In the meantime, I was becoming more concerned about Mother's safety living alone. I'd heard reported cases of persons wandering away, getting lost, and being in danger. Mother hadn't started wandering but there was always a first time. Even with Joyce's friendly help I was running myself ragged every day, going to and from the office and then back to Mother's.

I felt it was never going end. I began to feel that I was living in a time warp and Joyce was one of those angels walking around on earth. She spelled me, talked to me when I needed comforting and listened when I needed to express my frustrations.

With Joyce's assistance, I was able to slow down, catch my breath and tread water for a while. I realized that I didn't need to shoulder the burden of Mother's worsening condition by myself. Joyce was a friend when I needed her.

In those in-between moments, when I was able to get off the merry-go-round and think about the situation at hand, I realized with clearer awareness that we can only do what we can and only one day at a time.

Selfishly, I longed for our distant past. I remember Mother lying on her bed at her home on Chowen Avenue South. She loved the porch adjacent to her bedroom. She would open the French doors, allowing the fragrant night air to waft in.

Fresh air and the sound of crickets under the breezeway were a soothing addition to those quiet moments when all seemed perfect in her world. Reading by a small lamp at her bedside, Mother would slip into the plot of an intriguing mystery. And at her side her cat Chessie, languidly stretching, would purr with contentment and fall asleep.

A Bandage, Please!   9

M other was no longer an independent woman. Her world had turned upside down. She had fought to maintain control. Now she was losing the fight. She must have felt lonely and frightened. Mother now had no anchor, equilibrium or point of reference. Just getting through the day was a challenge for her.

She no longer occupied herself with her projects. She didn't have a job to go to, no partner to share with, few friends to socialize with, and she didn't care enough about eating to fix a meal.

Mother had been a voracious reader but new books sat unread.

All her life, her writing was a means of unleashing her soul. Now her journals lay closed, her typewriter unused. Her magnificent spirit was waning with each passing day.

I watched her losing her motivation to participate in life. She couldn't relate to the world around her, I observed grimly.

Coping with the uncertainty of Mother's existence I was losing my own equilibrium. I never knew what to expect.

I would find her in clothes that she had worn for several days in a row. She was not bathing or even grooming herself. Her apartment was becoming filthy and her refrigerator held little. I questioned her one evening when she appeared to be light-headed from lack of nourishment.

"Mom, what did you eat today?" She looked vacantly at me and shrugged.

"I think I had an orange and maybe some yogurt." I could see that there wasn't much to choose from as I looked through her cupboards and then the refrigerator.

"Mom, you can't survive on yogurt." She sa down in a nearby chair, staring straight ahead.

"I'm ok. I wasn't hungry, really."

Sometimes she would drift from one side of the room to the other when I spoke to her. She rarely left her building but when she did, she wandered around the complex, preferring to stay close to home rather than drive her car. One of the characteristics of the disease in the early stage is that that the stricken party constantly needs reassurance and restlessly wanders or paces out of the need to physically vent frustration.

She napped during the day and wouldn't pick up the phone when it rang. She rarely exercised anymore. She would take a walk around the nature trail in the back of her building if someone accompanied her. She left open cans of cat food out to spoil and forgot to change Chessie's litter box for days on end.

Because her judgment was impaired, it became unsafe for Mother to be alone. I was working full time and could not control what might happen in my absence.

Fortunately, she lived halfway between my home and the office so I could look in on her everyday. However, I felt I was on a time treadmill with no relief or break in the momentum of my existence.

Then in October of 1991, two months after Mother's diagnosis, an opportunity arrived. In truth, it couldn't solve the situation but it would provide temporary relief. I needed more help with Mother, and I wasn't sure how to find that assistance.

My twenty-three year old daughter Michele, a professional cook at the time, was injured and couldn't work. This meant she could not keep her apartment. After discussing her situation, I approached Mother to suggest that perhaps a roommate would be a good idea.

In a lucid moment Mother understood her granddaughter's predicament. "It's fine with me, Chris, as long as Michele abides by my rules." Even though she knew she had Alzheimer's, Mother was not aware of her growing confusion. She would fade in and out and was happy to have company, especially her granddaughter. Michele moved in on October 30, 1991.

For a while the arrangement worked, at least for Mother. For Michele, it was a challenge. As the weeks wore on I could tell that she was in over her head trying to take care of her. It was an exhausting assignment. Mother was becoming less able to do even the simple tasks.

Michele cooked, bathed, and dressed Mother. She cleaned for her. She tried occupying her grandma by watching television with her or accompanying her on short walks. Sometimes she'd read to her from her own writing.

Mother couldn't stay focused very long and would follow Michele around the apartment asking the same questions over and over or repeating stories of the past. I wasn't sure how long Michele would be able to endure the repetitions, demands and pressures of the situation.

I continued to work on the legal angles with Skip. I had approached Mother about needing to have all the details of her care in place. Having worked for attorneys for ten years prior to her retirement, Mother recognized the value of having her affairs in order and was sometimes still lucid enough to take an active part in decisions. She wanted the truth and I didn't hold back unless the information became confusing to her. In that case, I would back off and wait for her mind to clear.

Mother continued her therapy sessions with Ellie Bisek. Michele and I would attend with her, trying to gain insight into her level of impairment.

"Hels, what day is it?" Ellie asked. "Who is the president of the United States?" Ellie tried to make a game of it by being playful in her questions. Mother couldn't remember that George

Bush was president. "How many toes do you have on each foot?" Again, Mother stared blankly around the room, not relating to the fact that she had toes. For her, the questions were meaningless and the answers were lost.

One afternoon, a little wail came out of Mother. She sank down on the sofa and buried her face in her hands. "Chris, why is this happening to me? I have always tried to do things right. Why is this happening?" I put my arms around her and held her firmly.

"Mom, I don't know why. I wish I could tell you, but I can't." The truth was that I didn't have a clue.

Sometimes she would cry and at other times she would bristle with impatience. I remember all the times I would get frustrated watching her frustration. Secretly, I wished she would just stop struggling and let go. In time it was apparent that I was the one who had to let go.

Mother's condition was getting to Michele. My daughter was irritable and occasionally lost her temper. She would leave the apartment when the pressure of the moment got to her. She was showing signs of depression. I was unsure from one minute to the next what to expect. The disease was not only consuming my mother, but it was driving a gulf between Michele and me. Both of us were bowing under the strain. We didn't have enough knowledge and skill as caregivers to deal with the emotional and psychological wear and tear of the disease.

Alzheimer's Disease robs its victims of their cognitive ability, functions, and personality. Mother was becoming unable to discern where she was or what time and day it was. She was unable to function. Her life was disappearing before our eyes. And saddest of all, she was turning into a person neither Michele nor I knew.

It was painfully obvious we needed professional support. I began to investigate possible resources. We were on the same journey together, but the question in both of our minds was "Where do we go from here?"

Brief Sanity 10

T he realization hit all at once. I could no longer deal with the challenges of Mother's illness on my own, so I starting looking for information and help.

An acquaintance suggested calling an old friend of hers, Barbara Holmquist. She had been a family caregiver for her father who had the disease for eight years. I dialed her number and introduced myself.

"Hello Barbara, I'm Chris Winter. Isabel suggested I call. I understand your father had Alzheimer's." I heard her sigh.

"Yes, Dad had it. When he died I made a private pact with myself that I would help anyone I could facing the disease!" She sounded like someone who had survived a war. She recommended the Alzheimer's Association. I immediately called the Minnesota-Dakotas Chapter, requesting information. Within two days I had a lengthy list of all the support groups in the state of Minnesota. Several groups met in the Twin Cities area.

I began to attend at least three meetings a month, taking Michele with me. When I picked her up at the apartment, Mother was full of questions. "Where are you going? Can I come?" She couldn't understand why we were going somewhere without her. She despised being left alone and in her restless condition, wanted to tag along.

I knew that this was inappropriate. The meeting was geared to family caregivers, not the afflicted. We reassured her and left her at home.

The Alzheimer's Association eventually developed a group for those in the early stages of the disease, but at the time there was nothing available for Mother. As fearful and as lonely as she was, she would have benefited from meeting others like herself, with whom to share her feelings.

Attending a meeting was like being thrown a lifeline when your ship is sinking. Many days I felt like I was on the deck of the Titanic and there was no room available in the last lifeboat. I felt like I was alone floundering, drowning in despair, and then a light of commonality appeared in the darkness.

Sharing at these support groups pulled me out of the ocean of fear and ignorance. It reminded me of what I'd heard about Alcoholics Anonymous and other support for survival groups.

Time and time again, I heard stories of adult children dealing with decisions as their family roles reversed. It was odd and unnerving after spending a lifetime as the offspring. Our society does not prepare us for this parental role.

The adult children support group addressed all concerns that offspring had regarding their stricken parents. The attendees, some being their parents' only children, shared their concerns regarding decision-making without the support of other family members. Others who were siblings faced the conflicts of differing opinions.

In some cases, their parents had been together for years and one parent was afflicted; the other wanted to take care of his or her partner in spite of the tremendous burden. Such a parent partner, either a husband or wife, often refused help from their grown children. A struggle would ensue. The adult children would stand by, trying not to interfere, hurt their parents' pride or show disrespect. The caregiving would exhaust the caregiving parent who then became ill. Being ill and trying to care for a stricken partner is impossible. Unless witnessed day to day, it's hard for others to notice, let alone understand what caregivers are going through.

Group participation was comforting as well as enlightening. I felt as though I was part of a community confronting an unbeatable adversary. The facilitators were helpful and informative.

We learned that one must be able to accept each change and grieve for each loss in order to move on and prepare for the next level of deterioration. The devious characteristics of the disease became more familiar as time went on. Like others attending local Alzheimer's support groups, I began to adopt the philosophy of the Twelve Steps of Alcoholics Anonymous, scaling down my life to one day at a time. And as the disease progressed and Mother worsened, it then became a moment at a time.

I began to look forward to the meetings, sharing my experiences and supporting those who needed a boost. Our combined knowledge and information strengthened our group. Within one two-hour meeting, a person could learn about legal strategies, home care, behaviors associated with the disease, medical assistance, and the logistics of how and when to place a loved one in a nursing facility.

It was an enlightening and enriching experience to attend other types of Alzheimer's support groups in the metro area as well. I met individuals from all walks of life, religions, economic levels and races at these meetings. As we interacted we soon learned that we all shared the same common denominator, Alzheimer's.

Newcomers would arrive, watch and listen silently as the group shared. I could see wide eyes filled with pain and fear as I glanced around the table. The newcomers were silent for the first few meetings until they were comfortable enough to share their stories.

The old-timers had been on the journey for a while. You could see the acceptance, calm and resolution in their eyes as they came month after month. They had become very adept at polishing their swords and doing battle with the unpredictability of the disease.

At the adult children meeting, I met individuals who had a parent attending the spousal support group down the hall. The role of spouse has different challenges regarding the disease distinct from the adult child's issues, and it merited separate meetings to ensure the concerns of each family member were addressed.

Of all the various support groups I attended, I found the adult children support group the most helpful. We were all trying to do the right thing for our parents and found it was lonely. But the loneliness abated when we shared our stories. You could see the growth of individuals.

The routine was somewhat the same from meeting to meeting. We would gather around a large table. There was always fresh coffee and homemade cookies or some other snack. Julie Nygren, a staff facilitator, greeted us and had us take turns introducing ourselves. Julie, a former nurse practitioner, had lost her father to the disease, which carried a lot of impact. She was someone who had experienced and survived the rigors of the disease first hand. It was comforting to hear her story. The balm of such instant credibility cannot be replaced by written information.

Julie valued our experiences and encouraged us to share as much as possible. Our experience and insight was encouraging to others just starting this journey. The tremendous burden of the illness was shrunk, if only momentarily, when we shared with others. It became a proactive exchange that bred insight and even humor.

I became a substitute facilitator for our adult children group. It was a great opportunity to discover which issues were of primary concern, give to others, learn effective leadership, and continue healing. I also became a volunteer speaker for the Alzheimer's Association addressing family groups at nursing homes, churches and other civic organizations. The question and answer period following a talk challenged me, and I had to learn to provide statistical facts and materials to back up my statements. But it was my personal experience that brought the most attention from listeners. I became aware of the tremendous need in the public at large for information and support.

Looking back, I found strength in the interaction with others. I found a fellowship and commitment unmatched in its strength and purpose compared to any other experience I ever had before or since.

Interaction in support groups strengthened me to see Mother through her journey. This experience made decisions clearer and easier. I refused to be a pawn to the disease. I refused to be brought to my knees. I was swimming more efficiently. The sea had become less intimidating. Or at least I chose to think so for the moment.

She Wrote   11

A fter the disease struck, the most heartbreaking loss to me was Mother's ability to communicate. She was born with an extraordinary ability to verbalize and write. For as long as I can remember, she often remarked that she came from a family of writers.

Her grandfather Oscar had an amazing facility for words. In his later years, following the death of his beloved wife Jenny, Mother would often visit him, and they would share ideas and exchange writing pieces. She wanted to emulate him.

My great-grandfather Oscar was ethical as well as practical, being of the old school in which sound judgment was key to how one survived in the world. Occasionally, he gave Mother advice, but only when she asked for it. His opinions were important to her and he never infringed on her right to experience life on her terms. He told her, "Helen, any man who would ask you to compromise your principles is not worthy of you and is not your friend!"

His wisdom extended to his guidance in writing. Most of his work was poetry and he shared his favorite pieces with her. He wrote about nature as it related to his world and his personal experiences. He wrote a poem titled *My Garden*, and gave it to Mother. She kept it in a special frame hanging on her bedroom wall for years.

Mother loved writing poetry and developed a knack for it. Her older brother Channing also wrote, expressing himself through letters. It became apparent that somewhere in the family tree, the gene for the love of words took root.

Her writing ability served her well. Mother was always able to make a living, amuse herself during difficult moments and bring enjoyment to others who read her essays and poems. When I read her work, I discovered candor, humor, philosophy and wit in her ideas.

When she retired in 1984, she bought her electric typewriter from the company. She could now write on her own time and had the luxury of setting her own pace instead of being subjected to job pressures and the rigors of writing the legalese contained in lawyer's briefs.

She shared her many creations with me. I loved her witty style. Her colorful descriptions of ordinary subjects made them extraordinary and poignant. Her unique talent for words had been evident for as long as I could remember.

Then her early post-retirement writing which had been so prolific turned into occasional correspondence or typed notes on cards for her kitchen file. It dawned on me that Mother was writing less and less.

I could only guess why Mother's love of words had turned into a chore. To inspire and spur her on, I bought her one of my favorite books on the process, Natalie Goldberg's *Writing Down The Bones*. I had devoured every word of the book and found the author's insight and experience helpful with my own budding interest in writing.

Mother left the book on the shelf, and never opened it in spite of my enthusiastic endorsement.

Now that I look back, I realize that the gradual change in her attitude began with the move from Chowen Avenue. As time went on and the disease was claiming her, she could not do it. She had begun having trouble comprehending the written word. Her personal reservoir of ideas was emptying as her confusion started taking hold. When I discovered that she couldn't even write a check, I knew it would have been impossible for her to process an idea into even a short writing piece.

Concurrent with her abandonment of writing, her love of reading also began to wane. Mother had always been an avid reader and could finish a book overnight if it held her interest. At one time I browsed through bookstores, occasionally finding books that would interest Mother. Now she seemed indifferent. I began to suspect that she had a problem with alcohol.

She had been a party girl with Eddie and had learned to drink socially. When Eddie died, and the partying stopped, she continued to keep a bottle of brandy under her kitchen sink and would drink by herself in the evening.

Once, while she was still living in her former home, Mother confessed to me that she had an incredible urge for a drink at ten in the morning. The need for the drink at that hour of the day so terrified her that she left the house and walked around Lake Calhoun, over three miles in circumference, until the urge passed.

She never mentioned alcohol in that context again. However, the custom continued in her apartment.

Mother once told me what Eddie had said to her when he was dying. "Please, Mama, don't drink alone." I felt saddened at the memory of his request. It was as though she was desperately trying to hang on to the party days. She no longer had Eddie to share them with so drinking was an empty indulgence.

She also was becoming noticeably indifferent to other things that previously brought her delight. Mother even stopped reading her daily newspaper, a pastime she had engaged in for years.

In the old days, on Sunday morning she and Eddie would put on a pot of coffee and read the newspaper front to back, discussing news developments and laughing over the comics. The want ads were discarded and the obituaries held little interest. Now, nothing in the paper drew her interest. Nothing drew her interest at all. The fact was my outgoing mother was withdrawing from the world she once thrived in.

The creative, facile woman Helen Winter LaCaze was gone. Lost forever were the unique and clever ideas she spawned from her head and heart and put to paper. Her insight was obliterated, her wit silenced, and her bigger-than-life personality imprisoned by a tyrant. More and more, I felt the gravity of her fate: Mother would never escape.

Definite Diversions 12

Gradually, I began to accept Mother's fate and make peace with her destiny. Her present state of mind was the antithesis of the mind belonging to Helen Winter, the take-charge individual I had known and by whom I was raised.

The mother I knew was always thinking, reasoning, planning ways to provide us with a decent lifestyle, even when the pickings were lean. She could stretch a dollar better than anyone I ever met. She would find creative ways to balance the budget, prioritizing that which was most important to our daily scheme of living, often going without treats for herself in order to provide something special for me. She never showed regret as a result of her choices, necessary or not. She was unselfish in everything she did.

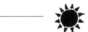

I remember so vividly her effort to put together funds so that she could give me a gift trip for graduation from high school on her salary. With my last year in high school coming to an end, she answered an ad by a local author who needed a final draft of her novel typed. Mother rented a typewriter in order to work evenings at home. She had a demanding boss at the time and she would often arrive home following a hellish day at the office bone-weary and in need of sustenance as well as relaxation. Instead, she hurriedly changed her clothes, grabbed a morsel, and typed well into the night.

When the author arrived in her shiny black Thunderbird toting her manuscript, my seventeen-year-old eyes drank in an eccentric woman of intrigue. She swept into our apartment in black from head to toe, a cape accenting her wide shoulders. Her enormous sunglasses concealed eyes lined in kohl reminiscent of Cleopatra. Her pile of hair was pulled tidy in a bun at the nape of her neck, and as she spoke in hoarse whiskey-coated whispers, her cigarette smoke wound in snake-like curls around her face. After going over her instructions with Mother, she made her exit with the panache of a cavalier, her cape the last visible evidence of her presence.

The novel was set aboard an ocean liner. It was apparently quite erotic but Mother never revealed the contents to my innocent ears. Later she confessed to me that as she was typing, the sexual details caused her to type faster, making it difficult to keep up with her own fingers. Each week the mystery woman returned with additional pages that Mother gleefully accepted, knowing she was in for a treat.

When the job was completed, Mother purchased two round-trip train tickets to California.

"Chris, we're going to visit Dale and Trudy," she announced. This vacation was a very special way of marking the closure of high school for me. Uncle Dale and Aunt Trudy were two of my favorite relatives.

Mother was giddy with excitement when she returned from work that day. As she was telling me details of the trip, she whirled around the room and hummed her favorite tune "On The Sunny Side Of The Street." Her devotion and effort to make it happen touches me to this day.

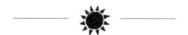

Now there was no consistency in Mother's behavior and it was becoming clear that she was too seriously handicapped to meet her daily living needs. I tried to keep her active and engaged in activities that were realistic and not beyond her understanding, providing as much interaction as possible. This took considerable guessing. I was never sure what she understood but her frustration often manifested in Mother's pacing around her apartment. At other times, she would repeat the same questions over and over, a behavior that proved to be frustrating as well as disquieting.

I was stumbling in a very dark room, bumping into every conceivable obstacle unable to find the light switch. There wasn't one.

Michele and I tried to keep Mother's routine as normal as possible. Outings provided a change of environment and a distraction for her.

We took drives to the outskirts of the Twin Cities metro area hoping that unfamiliar landscapes would hold Mother's interest.

We found restaurants we hadn't tried before.

We went to a lot of movies. This activity appeared to hold her interest. I tried selecting comedies, animated features and simple plot lines.

On one occasion, Michele and I took her to see the film *The Babe*, the story of Babe Ruth starring John Goodman. During this period Mother was becoming increasingly anxious about her bladder control. We no sooner got settled in our seats then she, in an anxious whisper, muttered, "Chrissy, I need to go to the bathroom." We were seated in a stadium-type theatre and had to traipse up and down the steps. Michele and I took turns taking her to the restroom.

I knew that Mother was frightened each time she felt the urge. Her agitation grew, bringing her close to tears. Distracted and unable to watch the film because of the interruptions, I had reached my threshold of irritation. "Again? You have to go again?" I couldn't tell if these anxious requests were false alarms or if she had a genuine need to relieve herself. Later I felt guilty and regretted my attitude. Mother couldn't help herself.

Another afternoon, I took her to see a Goldie Hawn film. Mother had always enjoyed any movie with Goldie, so I felt reasonably certain that she would enjoy the film.

After a half-hour of viewing, I felt the familiar tug on my sleeve. "Chrissy, I have to go to the bathroom. Would you please take me?" Once she was in the stall, I stood by waiting. After hearing sighs and mutterings from behind the door, she emerged, and staring straight ahead, wandered over to the sink, turned on the faucet and washed and dried her hands. When she finished, she turned to me with a bewildered look on her face and handed me the crumpled piece of paper towel.

"Chris, I don't know what is happening, I don't understand any of this." I studied her for a moment trying to understand what she was getting at.

"What don't you understand, Mom?" She was fidgeting now and inching her way to the door.

"The movie. Chrissy, what does it mean?" I followed her, assisting her by holding the door open as we went out into the lobby.

"Well, the star of the movie is Goldie Hawn. You remember Goldie Hawn, don't you?"

"Who's Goldie Hawn?" I felt an inner shudder and decided to forego the explanation. Instead, I walked her out of the theatre, as my stomach churned in a wave of indigestion, and emotional distress. We were quiet as I drove her home. No more escape in movies.

Evenings became difficult. After a pleasant night out, we would return to her place and Michele and I would take turns getting Mother ready for bed. When I was there on a typical evening, Michele took the opportunity to go out with a friend or just slip away to her room to read or write poems, two of her favorite pastimes.

After Mother had brushed her teeth, I would turn on the TV to distract her before I departed for home. As I'd reached for my coat, she would begin to cry. "Chris, I don't want to sleep. I am afraid I won't wake up."

I reached for her and holding her in my arms, I tried soothing her fears by talking softly to her.

"Mom, don't worry, I'm here."

"Oh, Chrissy. I don't know what's happening to me. I am so scared."

"Mom, you're not alone. You'll never be alone as long as I'm around!"

She would start to relax. My jangled nerve endings were wearing thin as these evenings became more frequent. Her ramblings would include what little information she could convey. She had so few words at her command, and what she could use she would repeat. I would bite my tongue and try to distract her long enough to make an exit.

One afternoon, I found Mother in despair and Michele absent. I guessed that Michele was fed up with her grandma's continual pacing and repetitious questions and had taken off.

Mother tried repeatedly to explain that a strange man was in the apartment shouting at her. I couldn't figure out who the strange man was. Suddenly I realized she was referring to Michele, who wore jeans a lot and had a strong presence.

Mother was convinced the intruder was still there, so I went through the motions, checking all the closets and obviously failing to produce anyone. Mother seemed satisfied, so I gave her medication and left.

Thinking over what I had just witnessed, I realized that Mother was having a hallucination of sorts, a symptom associated with the disease.

I discovered that it was easier to go along with whatever reality Mother appeared to be in.

Later, I spoke to Michele, mentioning the incident. "Hels was very upset, Michele. She thought you were a man and your outburst frightened her."

"Mom, I was pissed off!"

"I understand your frustration, but instead of flying off the handle when she bugs you, just remember it is the disease talking, not Hels."

"That's real hard to do, Mom."

"I know, but try to remember that she is not purposely trying to get your goat, ok?"

"I'll try."

I smiled to myself thinking that Michele wasn't the only one who needed more patience. I needed to apply my own advice. It was so easy to fall into the trap of thinking Mother was trying to annoy me, but the truth is she couldn't help it. She was becoming less able to process even the most basic information. My mother's personality was eroding and a stranger was emerging.

During this time frame, my uncle Paul called to report that my uncle Hugh, Mother's oldest brother, had died of heart failure. He cautioned me to not tell Mother because in his words, "Sis will brood." I thought about his remark and decided to hold off mentioning Hugh's death. As the weeks went by, I felt guilty about my omission.

When I couldn't keep it to myself any longer, I told Michele what I was going to do. "I'm letting the cat out of the bag. I'm telling Hels about Hugh."

"I think you should, Mom."

"How about tonight when I come over?"

"Good idea."

Later, as we were getting Mother ready for bed, Michele and I sat down with her.

"Mom, I have some news for you. Your brother Hugh died."

I took a deep breath, glancing at Michele. Mother responded nonchalantly. "Really? Well what do you know? He wasn't in very good shape, was he?"

I was surprised at her response, yet I was relieved I had told her. She never mentioned Hugh again.

As the weeks passed, I felt like an ant pushing a boulder up a hill. The role of conservator put me at the helm physically and financially. When it became necessary to institutionalize her, I had to make decisions on her behalf. In a lucid moment Mother said, "I know all this is necessary, but it doesn't make it any easier."

And so began the process of turning herself over to someone else, something she had never done. Mother had always been a responsible individual. First she had taken care of all the finances in her first marriage to my father. After she divorced him, she raised me and took care of her mother Christina who had no social security or pension, supporting us on a secretary's salary.

When Mother remarried, she ended up handling finances once again. Her second husband was irresponsible and incapable of keeping steady employment, a situation that almost brought financial ruin. Mother's tenacity helped her through this bare-bones time and after divorcing him, she started over. During her marriage to Eddie they agreed at the start that she would handle the finances. He was a free-lance industrial painter and worked job to job. There was no consistency to his income. Some months they were flush and at other times money was tight. She was salaried and had learned to budget.

When Eddie became unable to work because of a disability, she supported both of them. She took charge once again. This was her niche.

Now, Mother's mounting dependency was hard to watch, but with the help of her doctor, various health care professionals, our attorney, and regular attendance at support group meetings, I remained moderately successful in staying one step ahead of the disease.

Hardest of all was the unpredictable behavior caused by the tightening grip of Alzheimer's. I had taken over Mother's life, and her life had taken over mine. I took her everywhere. Michele did not drive, so she would accompany me when Mother attended therapy sessions with Ellie Bisek. I took her to doctor's appointments and assisted Michele with Mother when I wasn't working.

Michele's arrangement with Mother was challenging her mental and physical health as well as my own.

I was the designated recreational director, keeping Mother busy and distracted. I had no life of my own outside of Mother's needs and my job.

I was also continually worried about Michele and how she was coping. I set my routine for each day according to what was required in those three areas. Feeling as though I was wearing thin, I imagined myself like a trampoline, stretched and waiting for the next hard development to come down on me and rebound away.

Unwound Knot   13

Mother's tenacity had gotten her through some challenging experiences all her life. Growing up with her, I saw how resilient she was. Whether it was taking on additional work to earn extra money or standing up for her rights when her employer was unreasonable in his demands, she never found any situation insurmountable. Making our meals stretch on a small food budget, or finding humor in a situation that would bring most folks to their knees, she was indomitable. She never backed down when her values were tested or someone tried to compromise her. She was practical and spoke the truth. This posture intimidated some.

Early in her copywriting career, Mother was one of several hostesses at a party in downtown Minneapolis sponsored by the ad agency where she worked. During the gathering a gentleman recently hired sought her company, striking up a conversation. As the evening was drawing to a close, the fellow offered to drive her home. It was late, and a typical Minnesota blizzard was engulfing the city.

At that time we lived in Hopkins, then a small community west of Minneapolis. Because the buses had stopped running for the night, she reluctantly accepted the ride but explained that it would be a tedious drive, given the weather.

As they left the downtown area, snow was falling rapidly and visibility was limited. The car wound around generous drifts and the main road began to disappear under the blowing snow.

Without warning, about two miles from home, the driver pulled over to the side of the road, and turned off the engine. Mother explained that they were nowhere near her place.

Sliding one arm around the back of her seat and the other around her waist he moved in to kiss her. Surprised, Mother gave him a shove so hard that he banged his head on the driver's door. He stared back at her with a look of indignation. Determined to score, he advanced again. He made another grab for her. She reached for her handbag and smacked him hard across the face.

Adrenaline pumping, Mother grabbed the door handle, pulled down and shoved it open, quickly stepping out of the car. The snow was drifting up past her knees but she slammed the door and ploughed through the drifts, never looking back.

She stopped only to remove her three-inch, sling-back heels and trudged on through the crunchy snow all the way home. Later, sharing this experience with me, she remembered being so charged up that snowy night, she never felt the cold even though she only had on nylons.

Now all that fight was gone. She could not discern what she needed to do or when to do it. Michele was having trouble trying to communicate with her. She tried walking her through a series of cues when certain chores needed attention but Mother couldn't process the connection between the cue and the chore.

The first time she agreed to let me help her with her finances, I went to her cabinet and located a brown folding file in which she kept all her important papers. I showed her what I was doing, and sometimes she would nod, acknowledging that she understood.

With Mother directly across from me, I sorted through her statements. I told her which bill I was paying as I wrote a check. She would stare at me passively and as the time ticked by, would get up and begin walking around her apartment, talking to her cat Chessie and pacing to and from her bedroom. She appeared to be in a trance.

As I took over her finances, she remained indifferent. I felt like a snoop of the first order but I soon recognized the necessity. She had a large balance in her checking account and had written only a few checks in the past months. Bills were overdue. When I mentioned it, Mother grinned and replied slyly, "Don't tell anyone how much money I have!" I immediately began to monitor all her bills and payments.

Daily I was finding clues of Mother's disheveled thinking. For example, I discovered lingerie tucked away in a drawer with the price tags still attached. It appeared that she had repeatedly been shopping, bringing home her purchases, tucking them away, and forgetting about them.

"Mom, what a beautiful slip. When did you buy it?" I ran my hands over the shiny satin fabric.

"I don't know. Is it mine?" She stared blankly as I held it up to her, marveling at the shade.

"It's a great color!" As I started to put it back, she took it and held it out to me.

"Do you want it?"

"No thanks, Mom. You keep it."

Putting the slip back in the drawer, I remembered her stories of surviving the lean Depression years. I couldn't imagine her going on shopping binges, buying items whether she needed them or not, and then forgetting her purchases. She had been a discerning shopper.

Michele and I both tried to help her when she seemed able to communicate with us, but increasingly she seemed unable to express her wants and needs. We had to be devious because she was a proud individual and didn't want to be pitied or patronized by anyone.

One Saturday morning, Mother's pride reared up when I arranged for a friend, Martha Schaefer, to take her to the screening of a new film. I told Mother and she appeared enthusiastic about going out, but she couldn't function without supervision. This meant that we would get her up and prepare her for the day ahead. Michele performed this function on weekdays. When I wasn't working, I would come over in the evenings and on the weekend.

This particular morning, as I helped Mother get ready, I saw Martha pull up in her car. I rushed to the closet, grabbed her coat and began to help her on with it. She was struggling to put her arm inside one of the sleeves. The maneuver was too much for her to handle. In a low, guttural voice she growled, "Chris, stop pushing!"

I stopped, shocked at her reaction. In my haste to help her on with her coat, I had pressured her. She became upset because in her confusion she could not cooperate fast enough with me. I learned a valuable lesson that morning. I needed to slow down and respond appropriately to Mother's diminished capacities.

We take so much for granted. Simple tasks become monumental to the person losing cognitive ability. Mother tried to conceal her malfunctioning when she was aware of it but she could no longer prepare a simple sandwich, find programs with her television remote control, read and understand simple directions, select appropriate clothing to wear, or find her way to the mailbox.

Once, when I stopped over, I found the cat in an agitated state, pacing and crying for its supper. I told Mother that Chessie needed to be fed. At first she got defensive, but later expressed relief that I had reminded her.

One day I noticed a foul odor coming from her kitchen cupboard. I discovered she had opened several cans of cat food, leaving them uncovered in the cabinet. Days went by and the stack of cans never seemed to dwindle. Sometimes I spotted the cat's dish filled to the brim with untouched dry food. Chessie's weight remained surprisingly stable.

When Michele tried to guide Mother through feeding Chessie, Mother got testy, insisting on doing it her way. Chessie didn't get brushed regularly and her fur began to mat and form clumps. Over time, the knots of fur were difficult to comb out. The litter box held barely enough litter to accommodate a day's use. Later, Chessie developed diabetes.

Several times over a period of months, Mother mentioned her sore gums. Always fastidious about her oral hygiene, she had healthy and beautiful teeth all her life. She never missed her twice-yearly check-ups, so I didn't think too much about these remarks.

One evening Mother appeared tired and asked to go to bed. I helped her get undressed and suggested she brush her teeth.

As she brushed, chunks of brown matter fell into the sink. Shocked, I realized that she was brushing a severely diseased set of teeth and gums. Her toothbrush looked as though it had scrubbed the floor. I could see how distressed she was and now her complaints of discomfort added up.

I thought back and realized she hadn't mentioned her dentist for a while. She had forgotten to go and gum disease had developed.

I called my dentist Kordie Reinhold and arranged a check-up for Mother. Kordie carefully examined her mouth, and as she finished, she put down her instrument and turned to me. "Christine, your mother has periodontal disease."

"How serious is it?"

"Severe enough that I recommend her teeth be extracted and replaced with a denture." Mother sat quietly, staring ahead, and seemed unaware of our conversation.

"How soon?" My mind was reeling.

"I recommend at your earliest convenience. When you're ready, I know an excellent oral surgeon. Rhonda Altom is thorough and very caring." Having been a patient of Kordie's for years, I knew she would steer me in the right direction.

"Thanks for seeing us on such short notice. We appreciate your time," I said. Without another word, Kordie reached over and hugged Mother. Tears filled my eyes as I caught her glance over Mother's shoulder. She nodded to me affirmatively and smiled with her characteristic gentleness.

Although I did not know it at that time, the surgery wouldn't take place for a few months because so much was happening from day to day. We were becoming jugglers of more and more balls, yet we dare not drop a single one.

Lost In Paradise   14

By now, Mother's past was slipping away from her, and a grim void laid ahead. As I looked back on her losses, I realized she would never be free again to travel as she had immediately after retirement.

I remember her change of heart in the fall of 1991. Her indecision regarding her annual winter trip to Hawaii to see her brother Paul had seemed strange. She had always been a woman who hated Minnesota winters so much that she would book her flight in October. She would talk of nothing else until her plane roared down the runway, lifting off and carrying her away to Hawaii. I now understood the change was typical of the on-set of the disease.

Mother's youngest, fun-loving brother Paul had transplanted his family to Hawaii in the mid-60s, looking for new career opportunities and a change from living in Boston. He quickly adapted to the lifestyle of the islands, never losing his enthusiasm for his paradise. It spilled over on his sister.

I flashed back to her 1990 departure. I remember driving her to the airport, and instead of dropping her at the door, I went into the terminal with her. From the moment we got there, she appeared confused. After the ticketing agent told her which concourse to go to and circled the gate number on her ticket folder, Mother fumbled with her ticket for a few seconds and then, with a frown on her face, she turned to me.

"Chrissy, what does she mean? Where am I to go?" I was surprised with her timidity and confusion. I took her ticket and pointed to the number the agent had written and circled.

"Mother, you have to go to the Gold Concourse." She stood still, looking all around her, unable to make a decision.

"Which way is that?" Her demeanor was puzzling but not alarming at the time.

"You see that sign over there? That's the way to your gate, Gate 10." I pointed the way, giving her a hug, and wished her a safe journey.

As I walked away, I happened to turn around and spotted her still standing where I had left her. She looked confused as the crowd moved around her. I left the terminal, forgetting the incident until one year later in the fall of 1991. It was obvious that she wasn't going to Oahu.

It was now clear why Mother hadn't arranged her trip. She couldn't remember how.

Now, a year later in January of 1992, three months had passed since Michele had moved in. She had done her best to take care of Mother, but the situation was taking its toll. It was time to give Michele a break.

Since it was obvious that Mother was not going to travel by herself, I decided to accompany her to Oahu to see her brother Paul. When I called my uncle Paul and told him we would like to come, he encouraged us to visit as soon as possible.

I went to Mother's travel agent and booked our flights. I enjoyed attending to all the details of our vacation, including the packing. I was enthusiastic, thinking about visiting our relatives. I did my best to remind Mother that we were going to Hawaii. She seemed pleased about the visit with Paul and his family.

I stayed over at her apartment the night before our departure to make sure everything was in order and to assist her in the morning. I was learning that haste is a no-no with individuals suffering dementia. I needed to allow enough time to get ready. Rushing past a cue before she had processed it would frustrate us both.

On the day of our trip, we got to the airport early to check in. It was a charter flight, so I wanted to beat the crowd and not have my mother standing around longer than necessary. We sat in the terminal lounge, drinking coffee and engaging in a wonderful conversation. Mother was alert and able to interact with me more than I had experienced in months. I was thrilled, feeling as though I had her back free of the disease. We were called to board and as we took off, I remembered her love of flying on a "the big bird." I will never know if she realized she was on a plane but Mother relaxed and the trip went very well.

I informed my uncle Paul and his family of Mother's condition in advance of our arrival. However, when he and my aunt picked us up at the airport, he stared in disbelief as she struggled through the first moments of conversation. She spoke in short sentences and was no longer the articulate woman Paul had known all his life. Although she recognized her brother right away, it took longer for her to recognize her sister-in-law Margaret whom she had known for over fifty years.

On previous trips, Mother stayed with Paul and Margaret at their home. They were now living in a cottage furnished by their daughter Andrea and their son-in-law, Robbie Bell. It was only a few feet from the main house that sat on an impressive piece of property including an Olympic-size pool and regulation tennis court. This new unfamiliar location only confused Mother more.

Mother had trouble remembering her great-niece Emily and great-nephew Davis. It was awkward for the kids. Their great-aunt was in a confused state, doddering and slow to respond. However, they were sweet and respectful and each greeted her warmly with hugs and kisses.

By late afternoon, Mother was visibly tired and anxious. While Mother rested, I unpacked before dinner. Our sleeping areas consisted of a room for her with a folding screen wall, separating her from the common room, where I would sleep on a convertible sofa.

My rest was complicated by my relatives' nocturnal television viewing. The set was just loud enough to keep me awake. They also had a large cat that roamed the house at night and was especially playful at bedtime. My attempts to sleep were frequently interrupted by a heavyweight pounce. The combination of late-night TV and kitty tricks made my nights challenging.

The first night, I listened for sounds of Mother in the next room. I showed her where the bathroom was before we retired, and left a light on so that she could find her way. In the early hours of the morning I was awakened by the sound of running water. In a groggy state, I tried to figure out its origin but couldn't.

In the morning I heard her stirring so I went to investigate. As I slid back the partition, I found her sitting up in bed, staring straight ahead. "Well, if it isn't Helen LaCaze! Good Morning!" I did a dancer's flourish with my hands to put her at ease. She responded with a big smile when she saw me standing there in a Gene Kelly pose.

"Hi, Chrissy!"

"Do you want to get up now?" She looked around the room trying to remember where she was.

"Sure," she responded as she climbed out of bed. I gave her a duster to put on. I saw a wastebasket, noticeably wet. Looking more closely, I understood that the running water I had heard in the night was the sound of Mother urinating. She had gotten up in the night attempting to find the bathroom.

Disoriented in a strange place, she improvised and relieved herself over the wastebasket. I was surprised, and yet I was grateful that she had been so resourceful under the circumstances. I thought to myself, "Good job, Mom!" When I told my uncle what happened, he shrugged it off saying, "Don't worry about it!" As it turned out, Mother never repeated her mistake during the visit.

After breakfast the next morning, Mother wanted to take a shower. The cottage was designed to accommodate Paul and Margaret's needs, including a large stall-type shower room with a built-in bench. I found this a helpful feature because Mother could sit while I shaved her legs. When I finished helping her shower, I dried her and helped her dress.

I was disappointed because the weather was unseasonably cool for Hawaii in February. Although I had packed clothing for tropical use, I had the foresight to include light jackets to wear until the afternoon sun warmed us. I selected Mother's clothes, again purposely choosing colors she loved. She preferred easy care fabrics in warm colors, especially red. I tried to shop the way she had, because Mother had taken pride in her appearance.

I missed the days when I would buy something to wear and Mother, admiring it, would hint until I gave it up. She would squeal with delight and accept the item, often remarking how pleased she was. There had been a bright red, short-waist wool jacket with padded shoulders that I had bought on sale at Saks Fifth Avenue in Chicago. It had been a steal at the sale price. Mother took one look at that fall jacket and hinted and hinted until I relinquished it. She was thrilled and wore it often, remarking that it was her favorite.

As our vacation unfolded, Mother began each morning refreshed and focused. However as the day wore on she became tired and was unable to participate with the group. While we reminisced as we looked through family photos and other treasured memorabilia, Mother began slipping into a fog. I was aware of this behavior having seen it many times over. However, the rest of the family was unfamiliar with her withdrawal, and as they got more involved in conversation, they forgot she was there. Her silence and non-participation only served to isolate her more.

Health care professionals refer to this behavior as "sun-downing." I heard the term in support meetings from those who had witnessed the behavior. I also read in *The 36 Hour Day* that sun downing is that time of day, usually in the late afternoon, when the brain tires. In some cases, individuals become agitated, combative, and restless. Others wander or become silent. A temporary remedy for Mother's fatigue was to si ggest a nap. If she was restless, insisting that she go to bed didr 't help. She would vacillate between lying motionless on the bed with her eyes wide open or wandering aimlessly.

I rented a vehicle for the week, giving us fl(xibility and independence. We enjoyed the freedom of freew heeling around the island at our whim. Mother enjoyed the daily adventure. Our routine was the same but it always seemed new and delightful to her.

"Mom, would you like to go to the beach today?"

"Oh Chrissy, I would love to!"

"Let's go!"

"Ok!"

We would get into the car and drive a few miles to the ocean. It was a pretty ride, along winding roads accented by breathtaking greenery rich in tropical blooms. Mother liked the fragrance of the flowers and the soft breezes that blew gently across her face as she leaned closer to the open window. The sun warmed her skin and the familiarity of the environment brought her momentary pleasure.

I found a lovely beach near a little fishing village and it became our regular hangout. We walked for miles, chatting as we strolled through the surf.

At these moments, I felt as though Mother was no longer imprisoned by her diseased mind. Out in the ocean was an island with a small mountain at its center, so perfect it reminded me of a movie set. The beauty of the island was a captivating eyeful as its summit rose out of the azure-colored water. Singing "Bali Hai" from the musical *South Pacific* seemed just right.

One afternoon as we walked through the surf, Mother started to giggle, then she nudged me, nodding her head in the direction

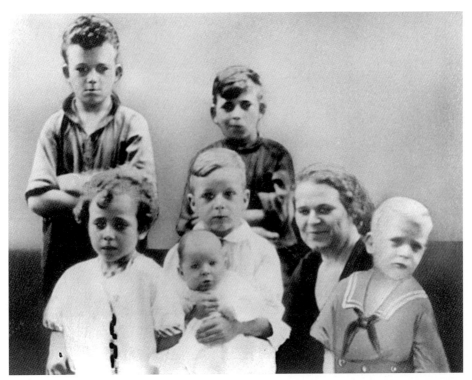

The Winter Family, c.1923. Rear, standing: Hugh, age 12; Channing, age 10; Front, seated: Helen, age 5; Paul, age 6 months; Vernon, age 7; Christina; age 34; Dale, age 3.

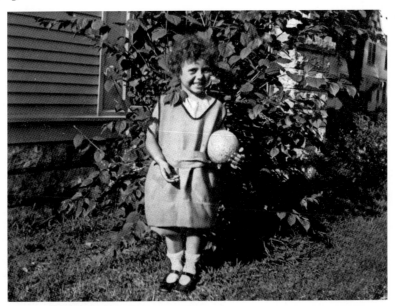

Helen in South Minneapolis, 1923.

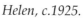

Helen, c.1925.

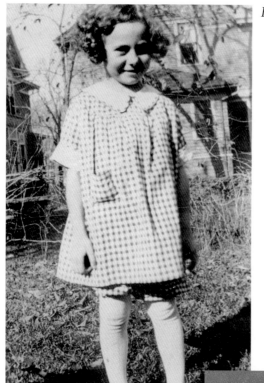

Helen Winter, age 18; West High School Class of 1936; Minneapolis.

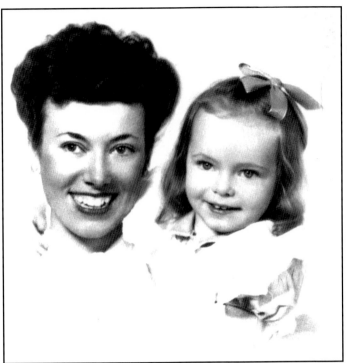

*Helen, age 26
and Christine,
age 3 c.1944.*

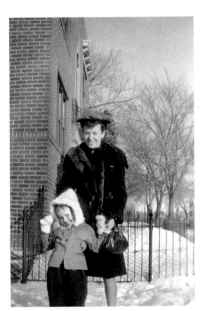

*Helen and Christine 1944;
Uptown–Minneapolis.*

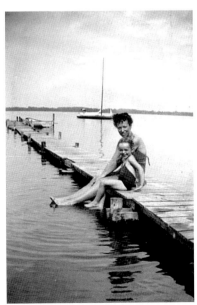

*Helen and Christine 1946;
Forest Lake, MN.*

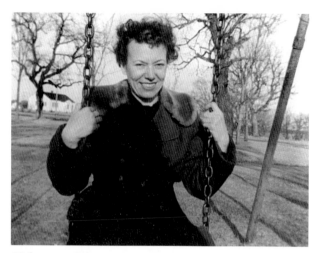

Helen, age 35.

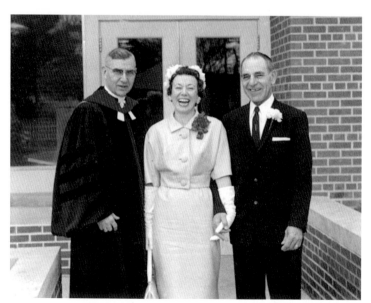

Reverend George Butters; Helen and Eddie LaCaze on their wedding day; April 22, 1961.

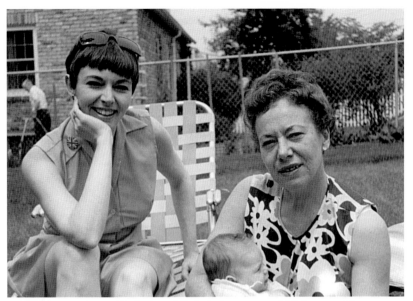

Three generations, Christine, Michele 3 mos., and Helen on Chowen Avenue, 1968.

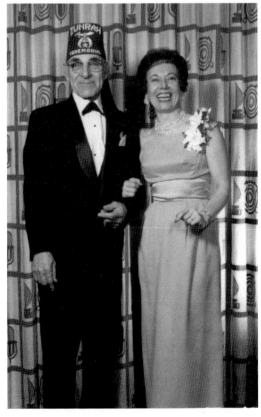

Helen and Eddie, Zuhrah Shrine Temple event, c.1970, Minneapolis.

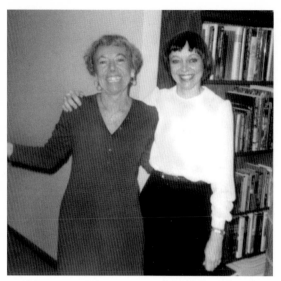

Hels and Chrissy, Detroit;
Christmas 1981.

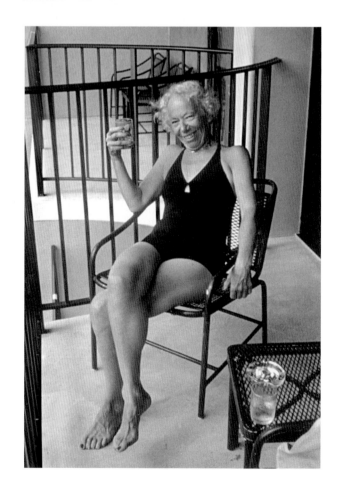

After retirement, Maui
vacation, 1985.

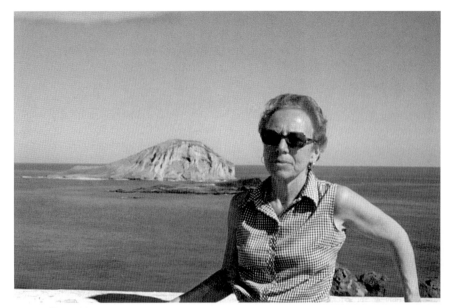

Hawaii, 1989.

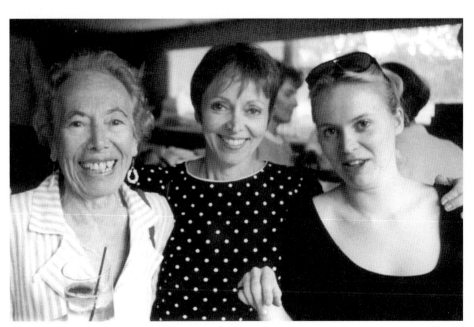

Hels, Chrissy, and Michele; September 1991.

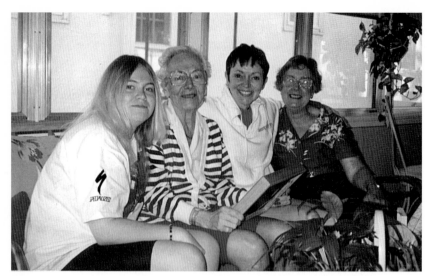

A visit to Martha's house. Left to right: Michele, Hels, Chrissy and Martha Schaefer, former neighbor during Chowen Ave. years, 1992.

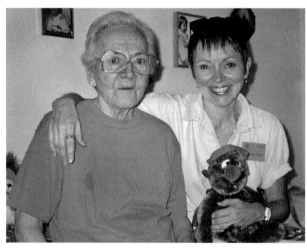

Hels and Chrissy, Luther Field Hall, September 1992.

of a couple passing us wearing thongs, a new fashion statement at the time. They were holding hands as they strolled, oblivious to the gaping tourists hanging out on the beach as they hung out of their thongs.

Mother was from the generation of the one-piece Jantzen swimsuit. Her figure was classic and the line of the suit had accented her firm and fit physique. Years before, she told me how she cultivated a summer tan and then, on a crowded day at the lake, walked the beach, strutting her stuff in a white, slightly transparent Jantzen. Mother relished the attention she got from male admirers, who whistled as she passed by. No wonder she found the near nudity amusing.

As we walked the dunes from the parking area to the beach one morning, Mother suddenly winced in pain. She jerked her leg and immediately limped. I had no idea what had caused her discomfort until I found a stinger in the sole of her foot, and removed it. She had evidently stepped on a wasp.

Soon we continued on our way, walking through the waves along the shore, the injury forgotten. I was again struck by how like a small child she had become, helpless and in need of constant protection as well as attention.

Our vacation activities included lunching at Waikiki, shopping in Kailua and sightseeing around the island. Neither of us had ever been to Pearl Harbor and while I found it a moving experience, Mother was not aware that we stood on the U.S.S. Arizona Memorial or the historical significance it had. She enjoyed the launch ride to and from the monument.

On return, we stopped for an ice cream cone, which appeared to be the highlight of her day. The past was lost to her and, like a child, only the moment mattered.

As time passed, Mother participated less and less with the family. Everyone tried to make the best of her obvious struggle by treating her normally. Davis and Emily tried to connect with their great-aunt Helen, showing her their rooms, their activities and introducing their friends. I was touched by their acceptance of her in spite of the obvious changes.

I learned by taking this trip, a person with Alzheimer's has difficulty in an unfamiliar environment. When a location is generic, like the beach, there is no pressure to remember. Staying with relatives one hasn't seen in some time in a new environment presents a challenge. Conversation is painstaking, and what was familiar in the past becomes foreign.

Our vacation week came to a close. Paul followed us to the airport where I returned the rental car.

As we said good-bye, I felt that this was the last time Mother and he would see each other. From my perspective, it was sad.

Most men of my uncle Paul's generation, especially men in our family, didn't show their emotions. Paul feigned nonchalance toward Mother, hugging her tightly and adding, "See you next year, Sis!" Giving me a sly wink, he got into his car and slowly drove away.

Mother had no idea where she was until I said, "Mom, we're at the airport. We're going home."

I suggested a snack before boarding, as we had to wait for over an hour before our plane's departure. As we ate, I made small talk trying to pass the time.

"Well, it's back to work tomorrow."

"Oh, where do you work?" I looked up from my sandwich thinking that Mother was kidding.

"Mom, you know that I'm with Nemer, Fieger and Associates, the same company I've been with for years!"

"You work for Nemer, Fieger and Associates? My daughter, Chris Winter, works there. Do you know her?" I sat there, not believing what I had just heard.

"Do I know her? Mom, I'm Chris Winter!"

"Well, I'll be a son-of-a-bitch!" Mother seemed to find my admission humorous and a flood of giggles followed. Her response gave me a bigger chill than if she had dumped a bucket of ice water over my head. I was floored and unable to comment any further on going back to work. We ate in silence as I tried to process what had just occurred.

There were no more surprises through check-in and seat assignment. We boarded the aircraft and pensively I took my seat next to Mother. We were seated in the center section of the huge plane.

I was exhausted, frustrated and melancholy. I just wanted to go to sleep and forget the previous week and our recent conversation, but my mind was flooded with questions. "Does she know who I am right now? Will I be a stranger again in a few minutes? Will we make it home ok? The week had been challenging beyond belief and not the vacation I had planned.

I put my seat back with the full intention of trying to sleep during the flight home. I purchased a headset so that Mother could watch the featured movie, hoping it would keep her occupied. My idea didn't work.

Just as I started to doze off, she leaned in and whispered, "Chrissy, I have to go to the bathroom." I unbuckled our seat belts, helped her across the row, and lead her up the long, narrow aisle to the restroom. I urged her to leave the door unlocked as I waited. When she had finished, we returned to our seats. Once I got Mother settled, I tried to nap again. A few minutes passed, and again I heard her plaintive request that required another trip up the aisle. Napping on this flight was not in the cards.

The trip going over to Hawaii had been such a breeze. Mother was relaxed and easy to travel with. She hadn't exhibited anxiety over her bladder control. In contrast, the trip home was disquieting with her constant need to go to the restroom and her inability to recognize me at the airport. Why was there such a drastic change in her cognitive capacity in just one short week?

The long flight home gave me time to think.

I was starting to feel anger as my mind mulled over the incident prior to boarding. My chest began tightening as my frustration grew. I thought about the challenges ahead and the prospect of dealing with the no-win nature of Alzheimer's.

Taking care of Mother was getting to me. The more I dwelled on the situation, the more hopeless I felt.

Showing my frustration served no purpose. I would upset her and aggravate my feeling of guilt. I knew that Mother couldn't help herself. She was bewildered, disoriented, frightened, and in need of constant supervision.

As a result of my own reality check, I began to calm down. Mother finally dozed off and I relaxed for the duration of the trip.

After what seemed like the longest flight in history we landed in the Twin Cities. My cousin Greg Winter met us at the terminal and drove us to Mother's apartment.

Michele was waiting when we arrived. She guessed my mood with just one look at me. "Tough week, Mom?" I smiled at her remark and obvious attempt to humor me.

The trip had been humbling. Now I fully understood what Michele was going through. I appreciated her more than ever. I took her by the shoulders and looking directly into her eyes said, " Thanks for hanging in, Michele." I felt such gratitude after my experience in Hawaii. I had briefly walked in the shoes of a true hero, a full-time caregiver.

May Day! 15

M other was bright, communicative, and witty before the onset of her dementia, and though afterward she struggled, she continued to have occasional moments of lucidity. At times she engaged in conversation. Her great nephew Michael Winter, a philosophy major at St. Thomas University at the time, was someone Mother enjoyed conversing with. She found his major fascinating. She thought he was special and was immensely proud of him.

She was also fond of Jill, Michael's sister. Jill is not only bright but also extremely independent, a trait Mother recognized they shared.

She also shared special relationships with all three of her brother Vernon's adult children; Jeffrey, Michael and Jill's father; Gregory, Jeff's younger brother; and their sister Lucinda, ten years younger than Gregory. Seeing them grow up over the years, Mother watched them develop into principled, talented and unique individuals.

When I told them of Mother's condition, they found it hard to believe, indicating they thought I must be mistaken. This doubting or denial was frustrating for my daughter and me. We began to resent what appeared at the time to be a cavalier attitude.

Even close friends, who had known Mother for a number of years, could not relate to what was happening to her. As she dropped out they seemed to forget her. They did not witness her gradual deterioration day by day, week after week. In retrospect, I could hardly blame them for staying away. The illness' grip on

Mother was hard to watch as it tightened. Alzheimer's support groups kept us on track, and attending them regularly infused Michele and me with understanding and courage. With each passing week, there was a little bit less of Mother.

She drove her car less and less. She rarely even thought about leaving the house. When she did get behind the wheel, she put herself and everyone on the road in danger. I finally asked her not to drive.

Paying her monthly auto insurance when the bright red Ford sedan sat ignored in front of the apartment began to seem a waste of money. When she remembered that she owned a car, she seemed apathetic about it. I now believe that she was forgetting how to use it.

I approached her cautiously, one afternoon. " Mom, I would like your car keys."

"Why, Chris?" She appeared surprised by my request.

I tried to swallow but my throat was dry. I had thought it through carefully, rehearsing what I would say to her. I responded gently.

"Mom, you haven't driven your car for quite awhile. Please give me your keys."

"Please, Chris, can't I keep them just a little longer?"

At that moment, Mother looked helpless and small. Restricting her freedom and independence by taking away her car keys made me sick to my stomach and sad. The thought of grounding Mother, like some teenager who had just misbehaved and forfeited her driving privilege, was difficult but I stood my ground. I was leaving town for a few days and couldn't risk her being left on her own with a car at her disposal. She surrendered her keys and ironically promptly forgot all about it.

Now, my mother's days appeared interchangeable. Thursday could be Saturday and summer could be fall. She no longer had a routine, and soon she just gave up trying to figure out what to do. Alternatively she'd panic and launch an endless barrage of questions again.

"Chris, what day is it?"

"It's Monday, Mom."

"Where are you going?"

"I'm going to work. I'll be back later this afternoon."

"Please take me with you."

"I can't, Mom. You can stay with Michele, ok?

"Ok, Chrissy."

Later, when I suggested doing something Mother could enjoy, she would brighten, and the distraction was good for all concerned. Her fierce pride relaxed and a few minutes of peace followed.

Michele continued to keep Mother's apartment clean and in order. She went about the daily tasks of changing and laundering linens and cooking her meals. However, a discovery one morning while cleaning Mother's bedroom reduced her to such panic that she called the office to tell me what she had found.

"Mom, I can't believe it. Hels wet her clothes!" Michele had gone into Mother's closet to pick up a pile of clothes for washing, and in the corner of the closet were a few articles of urine-soaked clothing. Her discovery was proof of Mother's growing incontinence.

I had witnessed her hasty trips to the restroom in movie theatres, understood her repeated requests were just in case, and felt her anxiety over losing bladder control. Now she was having accidents that embarrassed her. Realizing what she had done, she hid the evidence.

"What should I do, Mom?" Michele was still pretty shaken as we talked about this development.

Taking a deep breath, I decided simple was best.

"Wash the clothes you found and put them back in her drawer."

"Are you sure Mom?"

"Absolutely." Honoring Mother's pride was still important to me.

On another occasion, Mother had gotten up in the night and mistook a small rattan chair in her bedroom for the commode. When we discovered the accident, we had to dispose of the chair. Mother was struggling unsuccessfully with one of her body's most basic functions. Whether it was fear, pride, or simply forgetting to ask for help, she clearly needed it.

As the months dragged on, I became concerned that Michele needed more breaks. Attending support groups brought occasional relief for us both, but living with Mother full time didn't allow Michele any time for herself. Mother's continual anxiety and restless behavior were depleting Michele's energy.

As Michele grew up, Mother had been her best friend and surrogate mom. She couldn't believe that her grandma was becoming so childlike. I received another call at the office.

"I'm really upset with Hels!"

"Why?"

"She constantly repeats herself and wanders all over the apartment."

"Michele, she can't help it. She really can't. It's the disease talking, sweetheart."

"I know Mom, but that's not Hels anymore!"

I understood Michele's justifiable frustration and ire only too well. I felt we were trying to climb an insurmountable mountain. We had reached a vertical cliff and had run out of rope!

We decided that it was time to put Mother in daycare for adults. Her world had become so small. A planned and structured setting would give her some activity and interaction with others. At daycare, no one judged or stigmatized those with the disease. Everyone there was struggling with similar challenges.

In one of my support groups a woman who was a full time caregiver of her husband told me that she had enrolled him at Altercare. "He really enjoys his visits there, and boy does it give me a break." I called Altercare and made an appointment to stop by.

It was owned and operated by two women who were professional caregivers. My first visit was very pleasant. The facility was bright and clean. There was artwork on display, created by the participants and the large room was decorated thematically, depending on the season or holiday at the time. The owners were kind, patient and upbeat as they interacted with the attendees, who seemed content and happy to be there.

After the interview and a tour of the center, I decided to enroll Mother. I arranged to drive her there two mornings a week and to pick her up on my way home from the office. I also applied to Metro Mobility, a public transportation service operated in the Twin Cities. Because it was a popular service for the immobilized and elderly, it took a few weeks to add Mother to the schedule. When Metro Mobility finally kicked in, I was grateful to cross that task off my list.

In the beginning, she was resistant and very confused, repeating the same questions morning after morning. "Chris where am I going? Where are you taking me?"

"Mom, you're going to a party."

"Chris, what day is it?"

"Today is Tuesday."

"Oh."

She repeated the same questions morning after morning. In time, her anxiety ceased. As she became more familiar with her

119

new surroundings and comfortable with the staff and other participants, she appeared to relax and enjoy the activity.

In time, we had to add two more days of structured recreation to Mother's week, which required selecting an additional facility. I was familiar with Walker Methodist Center because one of my first support groups met there. A few family caregivers at the meeting had loved ones in residence at Walker. It appeared to be another good fit for Mother. However, unlike Mother's participation at Altercare, she never adjusted to the Walker visits. She constantly complained.

"I don't like it there. I don't fit in!"

"What do you mean, Mom?"

"They are a bunch of old people."

"Oh?"

I laughed, but her momentary lucidity threw me. I realized that I couldn't be certain how much information she was taking in. Her reactions were as inconsistent as her comments.

Mother continued to go to daycare four days a week. Michele and I had a game plan worked out. We called it "Operation Hels."

Weekday mornings I arrived early, on the way to the office, and let myself into her apartment. Going directly to her room I would wake her and take her to the bathroom. I started the shower and helped her in. Mother followed my directions as I handed her the soap and washcloth. After she washed herself, I would measure out a small amount of shampoo and remind her how to apply it. She obeyed, and after she lathered her hair I helped her rinse. After turning off the spray, I guided her out of the tub to the bathmat. As she made an attempt to dry herself, I would slip into Michele's room and get her up. Michele was a heavy sleeper and sometimes it took a few attempts to wake her. Once she was up and moving, I returned to Mother and helped her to dress while Michele prepared her breakfast.

Welcome to Worship at

Trinity Community Church!

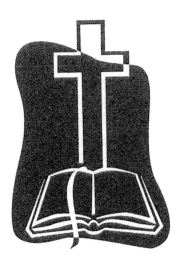

Welcome to our Worship Celebration
September 7, 2003

Today's Scripture: Colossians 1: 21 - 23

"Our Top Priority This Fall and Always"
Reverend Bruce D. Peterson, Senior Pastor

Trinity Church is a diverse gathering of friends who have discovered new
life through Jesus Christ and who seek to follow His guidance.

SERMON NOTES

TRINITY COMMUNITY CHURCH
234 Walpole Street, Norwood, MA, 02062
781-762-8408
www.trinitycommunitychurch.org

It was difficult for Mother to make any choices at this point, so I would select her outfits. I picked clothes that could be comfortably worn all day.

I was doing all her shopping. I chose fabrics that were easily washed and clothing that could be put on and removed with ease. At Target, I bought her a pair of tennis shoes with Velcro closures that proved to be practical. We never had to worry about her shoelaces becoming untied.

It was odd putting her through the same paces she had put me through when I was a child. She was like a child.

Once I had gotten her dressed, I left for the office, turning the rest of the operation over to Michele. She made sure Mother had a good breakfast. As she ate, Michele watched out the window for Metro Mobility to arrive and listened to the same questions every morning: "Where am I going? Why do I have to? How will I get there?"

Michele would respond simply: "Hels, you're going to a party. Someone is coming to pick you up. Don't worry."

This became a predictable daily experience for Michele, but for Mother each day was a new experience.

Role reversal was hard for me to adjust to. Mother had been so independent, I would never have presumed to know what she required in the past. Awkwardly, I felt I was overstepping my bounds but unfortunately "Operation Hels" was necessary. Trying to act in her best interest, I still felt I was betraying her. She was my best friend, my mother and my role model, and now here I was helping her to the bathroom and cleaning her up, intruding on her privacy.

I had heard of other people doing all these things for parents or loved ones when they became an invalid in some way, but I never dreamed I would become one of them. In reality, I knew I was watching Mother deteriorate, and there was nothing I could do except to ease her passage down unknown corridors.

Forced Decisions 16

Personal possessions became less important to Mother as the disease progressed. I began considering what needed to go but I found it difficult. I was intruding on her privacy again.

First, Mother's beloved cat Chessie needed a new home. In good conscience I could not surrender her to the Humane Society. She was over ten years old and would not be easy to place. She deserved a home where she would be welcomed and loved as an integral part of a family.

After a few inquiries my friends Carr and Marion Hagerman agreed to adopt her. They were animal lovers and already owned a dog and cat. Chessie would be a welcome addition to their home.

They took her to their vet for a routine check-up. The vet discovered that Chessie had diabetes. The disease had progressed to insulin dependence. Carr and Marion accepted the diagnosis and took her in as is. The cat lived another eight years, much to their amazement and mine.

Mother had loved her red Ford Fairmont, having driven it for twelve years. It was in mint condition but had been parked for months. The management of her apartment complex was threatening to remove it.

A friend knew someone needing a second car, and within two days we sold it. Mother signed over the title with little resistance. I don't believe she even knew that the transaction was about her car. She never even seemed to notice it was missing from in front of her building. We never mentioned it again.

May of 1992 arrived and with it, our court appearance to formalize my role as Mother's conservator. From initially meeting Skip to formulate this plan for Mother to this hearing, eight months had elapsed.

I tried to prepare Mother and continually reminded her of our court appearance. I didn't want any unnecessary surprises during the hearing. She was required to agree to my appointment as her conservator before a judge. It was a delicate matter. There was always a chance that she might forget her lines.

My bosses at the time were sympathetic and gave me the morning off. Michele got Mother ready by choosing business attire for her to wear. Wearing a tailored blazer and skirt, including a white shirt crisply accenting her appearance, she almost looked like the formidable businesswoman she had once been. How ironic that her disheveled mind didn't match her impeccable appearance.

Skip was business-like but cordial and greeted Mother warmly. First, we sat in one of many hearing rooms in the Government Center waiting for our petition to be read. Next, a court employee with a formal manner called me to the front of the room where I was sworn in.

From the witness stand I had a clear view of Skip and Mother sitting below the judge. As I answered the judge's questions, I looked down at my mother, sitting in the midst of strangers who were listening to personal details of her life. I wondered if she understood what was going on. I wasn't sure.

After the hearing, Mother and I sat in the Government Center plaza, drinking coffee and chatting. It was a beautiful spring day in downtown Minneapolis. Warmed by the sun, we watched the activity of a business day unfolding around us. I was distracted thinking about what had just taken place in the courtroom. It had been the last place I had ever expected to be with my mother. Mother glanced at me and shook her head sadly saying, "I wish things could be different, but I know they can't." Her independence had come to an end.

With my role as conservator in place, I began to plan placement for Mother to keep her safe in the care of professionals. The county's investigation of her income revealed that Mother had too many assets to qualify for in-home assistance. Michele had to get out. My daughter was not equipped emotionally or physically to handle Mother's increasing disability over such an extended period of time.

Mother's birthday was in June, less than a month away. The weather was so beautiful, that Michele and I decided to have a small picnic celebration behind her apartment building at one of the tables provided for residents. I bought Kentucky Fried Chicken with all the trimmings and invited our friend and Mother's neighbor Joyce. Joyce was still on occasion "Hels-sitting" when Michele and I needed to go somewhere.

It was a warm, summer day. We decorated the table in red, much to Mother's delight. The meal included a big birthday cake, and we lit the candles and sang "Happy Birthday."

Mother appeared pleased with all the attention and everyone had a great time, but in my heart I knew that this would be the last birthday she would celebrate at home. Michele knew too.

We did our best to distract ourselves with happier stories honoring Mother. We reminisced about life on Chowen and all the fun summers we had spent in Minnesota during my career as choreographer.

A marsh behind the apartment complex had a nature trail around it. Whenever we could we'd go for a walk along it in the greenery of early summer. We'd sing our way around the mile and half circumference of the trail. When she first moved into this apartment, Mother relished the activity. Lately, she did her best to keep up but toward the end of the hike she would be shuffling.

Mother's apartment complex provided a swimming pool for tenants. The weather was warm and inviting, and I encouraged Mother to swim. This activity had been a lifetime passion, and after she retired, she joined a local health club to swim. Only a few years ago she had never missed a day. I had tried to convince her to take a day off occasionally, but she wouldn't hear of it. Mother lost interest in swimming when her dementia set in, and had let her club membership lapse.

I bought new bathing suits for the three of us and Michele and I took Mother swimming. I reasoned that swimming would ease her anxiety, give her exercise, and relaxation. I wasn't sure if her affliction would endanger her, so we jumped into the pool with her and supervised her carefully.

When she swam in deep water, I reminded her to return to the shallow end. She'd remember my warning for a while, but inevitably she'd forget.

For a few weeks we continued our poolside vigil, but soon it was apparent that Mother had lost her stamina. I could see her becoming physically weaker. The look in her eyes as she struggled through her strokes was a warning that it was time for her to quit.

With each passing week, Mother was struggling more and more. She lived in a perpetual state of confusion.

For a while, going to daycare four days a week had filled Mother's need for structure and gave Michele some much-needed rest. However as time went on Mother would return home anxious, disoriented, and exhausted, creating additional stress on Michele. I tried to help by stopping by after work or asking Joyce to stop by.

"Chris, I'm so scared, please don't leave me," became a familiar plea each time I tried to leave and go home. Bone-weary from working at the office, I needed some time to recharge my own batteries. After a few minutes of calming persuasion, I would leave Mother with Michele, but I could see desperation in Michele's face too.

When I broached the subject, her eyes would fill with tears. She would shake her head, saying, "Mom I feel guilty, but I can't take much more of this." Sometimes she would even threaten to leave. I wouldn't have blamed her if she had. In our support group, we were constantly reminded of the toll on family caregiver's mental and physical health as the disease progresses. Mother's clock was ticking. Alarms were going off. The time was coming when we'd have to place her.

One workday morning, I received a call from Altercare. Mother had arrived perky and enthusiastic. However as time wore on, she became agitated and frightened and refused to participate in any of the activities. None of the persons she normally interacted with looked familiar. All were strangers, including the staff.

I called Michele to tell her that Mother would be home early. I took my break earlier than usual and went to pick her up. I found her curled up in a corner by herself. I approached her, speaking softly, "Mom, it's me, Chrissy." She immediately calmed down when she recognized me. Mother tried to tell me how she was feeling. As jumbled words tumbled out she grabbed me tightly. As I held her, I tried to make sense of the jumble. The only clear idea she could express was, "Chris, I want to go home!"

I helped her up, trying to speak calmly. "Mom, it's ok, I'm here. I'm going to take you home, ok?"

She hung on tightly and kept saying, "I want to go home, I want to go home," as we walked toward the door.

She was worn out when we returned to her apartment. The relief she must have felt was obvious. She began to relax, even smiling a little. We undressed her and helped her into bed. She fell asleep almost immediately. The final alarm had gone off. Michele and I exchanged a look of resignation. It was time to place her.

Plans for Peace 17

I n anticipation of Mother's inevitable placement, Michele and I had already started an intense search for the appropriate facility. We knew that this was going to be Mother's last home so the right selection was one of the most important decisions we'd make.

By investigating a number of care centers throughout May and June of 1992, I developed a gut-level feeling about each of them. They were not equal in terms of the level of care or staff experience.

Some facilities were not familiar with the challenges associated with dementia like Alzheimer's. In some cases all the residents regardless of ability or symptoms are placed in the same units. This is not appropriate for residents with dementia nor for those who have their faculties but are deteriorating physically.

Dementia residents must be in units that are locked. Staff members need special training to handle the problems associated with neurological mind disorders.

For me, placing Mother in a nursing home was akin emotionally to sentencing her to life in prison without parole. I know that this feeling was extreme, but in her final home, she had to be as secure and comfortable as possible. She deserved to be with professionals who had the training to deal with dementia, but also had their humanity in place. As I interviewed staff members of various facilities, I looked for certain qualities in their attitudes toward residents; courtesy, experience, kindness and respect were high on my list. Placing Mother in other hands, I was determined that she would receive the best and most appropriate care.

We narrowed the list to four facilities.

One facility was beautifully appointed with the newest equipment and plush décor sitting on a pastoral piece of land, but it would have been a long commute from either my home or office. Though the facility was physically beautiful, the staff seemed too businesslike and somewhat elitist.

Another was old, worn, in need of upgrading, and located in the inner city in a high-crime area. However, the administrator was kind and helpful, and the staff appeared respectful and interested in the residents.

A third facility was vast in size, and felt cold, reminding me of a compound that sprawled like a town. The administrator behaved like a high-pressure salesperson, more interested in our funds than our needs.

The fourth and most institutional-looking building put me off the minute I walked through the door. It had a hospital smell suggesting cleaning agents masking decay and illness. Staff responded to residents rudely or appeared indifferent to their needs.

Cost was an enormous factor in my decision. Until we could apply for medical assistance, I would be paying the entire monthly fee from Mother's income. Back in 1992, the cost of care ran from $2100 to $3500 a month, depending on which facility one chose. Making a good choice was crucial.

I decided on the second nursing home, Ebenezer Field Hall. It was an easy commute from my home or the office by a number of routes depending on time of day and traffic.

It was located in the inner city in a care-worn area but parking was convenient to the front door. It had a twenty-four hour surveillance system and a security escort available.

I toured the facility and talked extensively to the administrator. She was attentive to my concerns and very informative. As we visited, she led me to the occupational therapy center. Residents with dementia had created the art on display there. The display showed me how important it was at Ebenezer to preserve the personalities of those who created the work hanging there. I knew in an instant that this was the right home for my once-gifted and lively mother.

The administrator placed Mother on its waiting list and told us that there would be an opening for her anywhere from six weeks to six months. She explained that when Mother reached the top of the list, they would call us to see if we were ready to place her.

The next challenge was to prepare Mother to move. Mother had always feared nursing homes and refused to visit anyone residing in one. I believe this attitude was formed when she watched her own mother live out her last days in the throes of cancer in such a facility. Mother never forgot those visits to Grandma's tiny room. The hideous green color on the walls and the odor of sickness were indelible. The experience filled her with a dread of nursing homes.

Another negative experience occurred when we visited my aunt Kathryn Winter, Mother's brother Channing's widow. Kathryn had placed her failing mother in a local facility. She asked us to accompany her on a visit.

The building was old, the rooms were cramped and the stench of bodily functions and disinfectant permeated the air. After a brief visit, Mother wanted to leave, so we made our exit.

In the parking lot, she began to hyperventilate. "Chris, don't ever do this to me!" She was close to tears. I remember giving her a hug, but not being able to relate to her outburst. Now I was dreading doing to her what she feared so much.

Month after month I had attended the adult children support group. I heard family members sharing their trepidation over placing a loved one in someone else's hands. Siblings had difficulty agreeing on what course to take. Some found it agonizing to separate parents who had been together a lifetime.

As people shared, the scenario was curiously the same. Each expressed an immense feeling of guilt associated with removing a parent from the comfort and familiarity of home to a foreign environment. The adult offspring at meetings would shake their heads in despair. How could they make such a decision? How could they institutionalize a mother or father in a new environment, one in which he or she would have to adjust to total confinement and the care of strangers? These were our parents and now we had to make decisions for them in their best interest but, more often than not, against their wishes.

As an only child I made all the decisions. At times it was lonely but on the other hand, by contrast, I often observed debates between siblings deadlocked in disagreement, emotionally out of control, and paralyzed by the fear of confronting the parent caregiver. Whole families became emotionally drained as they struggled to make decisions.

Returning from Hawaii, Mother required more care than ever. It was as though the disease process had accelerated suddenly. We saw a more consistent decline. Michele and I got so stressed out that we developed bronchial infections, forcing us to slow down. In spite of being ill, we had to keep plugging away to keep ahead of unfolding developments. I craved rest and wanted to sleep away the weariness in my body and the wretched hurt in my soul.

The alarm clock would sound. Slowly I would get up and prepare myself for another day. During the week, I would go to my job on a busy switchboard and afterward visit with Mother. I returned home late in the evening and collapsed into a heap, drained physically and mentally. I was grateful for my weekends because I could sleep in a little before returning to Mother.

I discovered a way to relieve the pressure cooker build-up of emotions. After a visit with Mother that had been especially difficult, I'd drive home with the windows rolled up, yelling as loudly as I could. Or sobbing as the tears ran down my face, I would talk to my Higher Power. By the time I had arrived home, I was ready to face the next hurdle. These momentary outbursts also renewed my confidence that I was doing the very best I could and that was enough.

When my rage passed, my next thought was how to take better care of myself. A brisk walk, a call to a friend, or soaking in a warm bubble bath helped. Meditating on the good things in my life would also help put my current position in perspective. Mother's deterioration became more overt. She could no longer follow simple cues. Getting her dressed or helping her brush her teeth led to constant frustration. Michele was often in tears and called me at work just to vent. This was not always easy to handle given my responsibilities at the office, handling the switchboard and covering the front desk. I had to be cordial, energetic, enthusiastic, and upbeat to company staff, clients, vendors, and a variety of delivery people. Often I felt torn.

My employers at the time were Jim and June Fieger of Nemer, Fieger and Associates. The Fieger's motto had always been "family first." Whether it was for a doctor's appointment for Mother, a meeting with our lawyer, or handling small emergencies that came up, they never questioned my need to be excused.

Then, one day, Mother became too much to handle. A desperate call from Michele made it clear that we had to act. Frightened if she sensed she was on her own, Mother was following Michele everywhere she went in the apartment and constantly asked questions.

Michele couldn't even get the privacy she needed to use the bathroom. Mother kept calling out to her when the door was closed, unnerving her. I called the care facility to check on the waiting list and requested immediate placement. Mercifully it was only a matter of days before Ebenezer Field Hall had an opening for Mother. Her life in her apartment was over. My role as conservator was in place. Her finances were in order. The inevitable time for this change had arrived.

The Inevitable   18

Unlike many journeys where you have the option of turning back, there is no such option with Alzheimer's. Mother's moving day was July 11, 1992. I tried to prepare her. I hoped that some information regarding her move would stick. It was difficult to know what was getting through to her and what was lost.

I also busied myself with details. I gave notice to the manager of the apartment complex for the end of July. Her month-to-month agreement required a sixty-day notice. Since it was now the end of June, Michele agreed to stay to meet the sixty-day requirement and that satisfied the management.

In the meantime, my lawyer advised me to liquidate Mother's remaining funds to spend down to the county's asset limit of $3,000. With this amount of savings remaining, she would qualify for medical assistance; all of Mother's monthly income would be used for her care, and the county would supplement it as necessary. The irony was that she had worked diligently all her life for this nest egg, and while it would provide for her care, she wasn't aware of her success.

I bought Mother some comfortable new clothes that would be practical and Ebenezer provided me with name labels for each item.

I purchased a bright, floral comforter to liven up the sterile room. Mother would be taking a favorite lamp with a vibrant red base to provide light at her bedside.

I also took inventory of her stuffed animals, pals that had been with her for as long as I could remember. Mother loved her "big cats" as she called them, an impressive group of lions, tigers

135

and leopards. Her bed had been covered with them. I called them her "soft zoo."

Mother barely seemed to notice all this activity and wandered behind me as I moved from room to room choosing what she would take to Ebenezer. I think I was more uptight about the impending change than she was. I felt guilty and sad about having to place her in a "home." At the end of an evening, I would leave her apartment in tears.

I remember the day before the move to Ebenezer, a Friday. I had been hired at Nemer, Fieger and Associates four years earlier largely due to my friend and former theatre associate Joel Thom. He was vice president of promotions and publicity for the film division of the company. We had worked in community theatre productions and had developed a close relationship over the years. I had rented an apartment in his home, so we spent time together outside the office as well.

Joel had also developed a friendship with Mother through his association with me. He often reminisced about the good times he had with her over the years. Whether it was showing up during lunch hour, carrying a picnic hamper to share with her in the park across the street, or wining and dining her at a smart establishment along the Mississippi River, Joel was a devoted friend and was well aware of her Alzheimer's.

During the summer months, the Fiegers gave each employee half of Friday off every other week. This Friday was my turn to work through the afternoon. Staying focused on work was tough. In my mind I kept mulling over the details of the next day's move. I felt dizzy and overwhelmed. I needed to eat something. A fellow employee offered to get me some lunch, ordering a salad from a local deli.

After lunch, I began to feel queasy. Another worker took over the phones. Walking back along the hall to Joel's office and knocking on the open door, I stood silently, trying not to cave in. He glanced up from his work, a "what's going on?" look on his face. I was shaken and began to cry.

"Hon, what's wrong?" I stood there, crumpled, leaning on the frame of the door.

"Joel, I am losing it. I'm going to pieces."

He immediately got up from his desk and opened his arms to comfort me. He knew Mother was going into Ebenezer the next day. Burying my face in his shoulder and sobbing uncontrollably, I held onto him and he let me until I was ready to let go. He invited me to rest on his sofa for a couple of minutes while he covered the phones. The room was spinning as I sank onto the couch and put my feet up. "I have to get up, please God, help me!" Breathing slowly I began to calm down, and realized that the fear and the guilt in having to place Mother had made me physically ill.

Suddenly, I felt nauseous, so I struggled to my feet. Heading for the restroom, I entered the closest stall, and fell to my knees, retching. A few minutes passed. Slowly gaining my equilibrium, I returned to the front desk. Joel left only at my insistence as it was his turn to take the half of day off.

The workweek came to a close without further incident but a new lesson stayed with me. Fear and guilt could make me sick. Retching had not only released the physical sickness, but it also released my emotional torment. I finally accepted the fact that I had no choice but to place Mother.

Friday evening I picked up Mother, Michele and Joyce, and we went to dinner. Agreeing that it was pizza we wanted, we ate at a favorite restaurant in the neighborhood.

After finishing the meal, we walked to a nearby greenhouse. I bought plants for everyone, finding a special one for Mother. The plant leaves were pink, etched in green with polka dots, giving it a whimsical appearance. The whimsy of the plant masked my mood. I was really thinking Mother's time in the outside world was running out.

Suggesting to Mother that she should go to sleep as the evening had been a full one, Michele and I helped her change into her favorite robe made of red satin. Together we sat on the sofa, Mother sitting between us. Feeling very calm and clear of purpose, unlike my state of mind earlier in the day, I began explaining to her that she was moving in the morning.

I carefully told her what to expect. "Mom, you are moving in the morning. You are going to a new home at Ebenezer. You won't be alone and Michele and I will visit you every day. You will get all the things you need now."

She nodded slowly, and then she began to shake. I put my arm around her, trying to calm her, but her body shook even harder.

I could only guess that she understood and was terrified about what lay ahead for her. Some minutes passed and gradually her shaking subsided. She had exhausted herself and she needed sleep. Michele and I helped her to bed. We kissed her goodnight and she fell asleep immediately.

Now the course was set. Mother would be protected in a safe environment, monitored by nurses and aides who would never know her as we had. Strangers would control her, and we would become interactive spectators in her life. I already felt a let down, a loss.

Looking back, I realized that her life had begun to change forever when the first traces of Alzheimer's began. Nothing had been the same after that.

This Is Home?   19

S aturday, July 11, 1992 arrived. It was hard to believe that only a year had passed since I had confronted Mother with my concerns over her puzzling behavior. Eleven months had come and gone since her diagnosis. I could still hear Ellie Bisek's words as I turned them over in my mind. "Hels, you are in the early stages of Alzheimer's Disease. What do you think about this?"

I half-smiled at the memory of Mother's glib response, "I feel like going out and getting loaded, but I know it won't do any good." And today, Mother was moving into her new home at Ebenezer Field Hall.

When I arrived at Mother's apartment that morning, it was evident that Michele was feeling at loose ends. She shared her conflict about letting go of her role as Mother's caregiver. Her great love for and loyalty to her grandma made it all the more difficult for her to give up and give in to Mother's decline. But the progression and severity of Mother's disease made it impossible for Michele to continue in the role of family caregiver.

I knew it was going to be a difficult adjustment for her. She had become adept in caring for Mother in spite of her lack of training, but she also paid a price for her inexperience. Unlike the professional who works a shift and then goes home, Michele was with her around the clock and had become physically and mentally worn out. She had a fiercely protective attitude and was challenging me.

"Those people down at the nursing home better take good care of Hels."

"It's a given. They do the very best, just as you have, Michele."
She was growing feistier and very vocal as she continued.

"Well, they better!"

"Don't worry."

Because of the isolation the disease brings to the afflicted as
well as to the individual providing care day in, day out, Michele
was out of touch with her friends. They never stopped by or
called her anymore. She missed the challenge and creativity of
working for some of the top chefs in the Twin Cities, honing her
skills as a professional cook. She had come to the end of
providing all-consuming home care and it would force her to start
over professionally. She was apprehensive. I hugged her and
suggested we get on with it.

Because it was such a beautiful morning, I suggested the
three of us go for a walk. For me and for Michele, this was a
special event because Mother would never walk this trail again.
As we strolled the wetland, birds were evident everywhere along
the path as though they had come to say "goodbye." Melancholy,
I began singing Mother's favorite songs. Soon Michele joined me,
and then Mother began singing with us. Here we were, three
generations of women in one family singing and skipping around
the marsh. The walk came to an end too quickly. We left the path
and returned to the apartment.

With the car loaded, we helped Mother into the back seat,
rolled the windows down and drove down to Ebenezer Field
Hall. The charge nurse Leslie Hart met us. She was a short, pretty
brunette who bore a resemblance to Leslie Caron the French
dancing star of MGM musicals. She was gentle and kind as she
took Mother by the hand, leading her into the elevator.

We rode to the third floor, a secured area designated for
dementia residents. Leslie punched in the access code at the door
and we waited for it to open. Entering the lock-up for the first
time with Mother was an unnerving experience. All I could think
about was the prison-like feel.

Female residents filled the halls. They wandered bacl forth, vacant stares on their faces. Some appeared to be lo confused, while others aggressively paced up and down tne corridors walking to unknown destinations. Other residents used wheelchairs or walkers to get around. Their ages ranged from late fifty to ninety years.

Some of the older ladies, their hair neatly done, wore dresses accented by jewelry. Others had on bathrobes or sweats.

I smiled when I caught a look from a woman walking toward me. As she passed, she greeted me with an emphatic, "Hello, dear."

Another woman became combative as an aide tried to take her to the bathroom. She lashed out and shoved at the care worker, screaming four-letter expletives at her. I watched as another aide took over, calming the distressed individual. In that moment, I saw how caregivers here needed fortitude, patience and strength to handle their unique charges.

The whole staff worked in high gear, taking into account each detail of care needed. For them, it was business as usual. To the untrained like Michele and myself, handling each and every resident seemed like an overwhelming task.

We located Mother's private room a short distance from the common area that served as a dining hall. The tiny, dull beige space was long and narrow. A window at one end looked out on a courtyard. It needed a touch of fresh curtains. The floral comforter I bought would brighten it too.

In three years' time, Mother had gone from her private home and yard on a quiet, tree-lined street to the impersonal, transient environment of a multi-unit apartment complex to this miniscule, sterile room in a locked care facility. The contrast was a vortex of change with Mother caught in the middle, her surroundings diminishing out of her control.

I unpacked her belongings to help her get settled. Once again I had brought a hammer and some nails to hang up her favorite pictures, just as I had done the day she moved into her apartment. It was natural to assume that the photos would provide Mother with familiarity and comfort in her new surroundings. However, she was feeling lost in this strange new place.

She became cross and agitated repeating herself often. "Chris, what is this place? Why are we here? I'd like to go home."

I changed the subject. "Look, Mom. I brought your favorite stuffed animals. Here's Leroy the Lion. He wants to snuggle with you right here." I continued to add touches of home but the cramped space still looked like a hole in the wall. The stuffed cats did little to improve Mother's new surroundings.

Once I had unpacked her belongings, filling a small chest of drawers and a closet, I suggested that we go exploring. I asked Leslie, the charge nurse, if we could take a tour. She suggested we go to the seventh floor lounge where we would have a panoramic view of the city.

Getting off the elevator, Michele noticed a large birdcage strategically placed in a seating area. The cage was home to dozens of colorful finches that warbled and chirped filling the space with lovely song. We walked into a large area that had floor to ceiling windows all around the room. This was the facility's recreation area, serving as a chapel on Sunday mornings. There was a large, separate, glassed-in room used for care conferences, and enough space to host special events.

As we walked over to the windows to peer out at the view, I noticed Mother scowling. The look on her face said it all. With a tone of disgust she muttered, "I want to go home, now! I hate it here!" She seemed lucid enough and I could see that she was already unhappy.

Mistakenly, I tried to convince her that this was a nice place for her. "Mom, you are gonna love it once you get used to being here."

"How could you do this to me?"

I felt a wave of guilt pass through me as I responded to her lucid, pointed question. "Oh Mom, please, don't say that."

She turned her back to me and ignored any further pleas.

It was futile. What could I say? Emotions choked my throat. The more I tried, what Michele referred to as "tap dancing" through a difficult moment, the more disgusted Mother became.

We returned Mother to the third floor security unit and reassured her that we would return. Leslie's shift had ended, and a new charge nurse introduced herself to us.

Vera West was a veteran caregiver, an older woman with a pronounced British accent. Her manner was kind and respectful and she had a charming sense of humor. We heard she often sang residents' favorite songs, as suggested by their families.

Vera could sense how awkward we felt this first time, trying to leave Mother behind. We kept trying to distract her with trite conversation as we worked our way back to the security door.

"Why are you leaving me? I don't want to stay here!" Mother grabbed on to Michele's hand, holding tightly. I took Mother's other hand as we continued walking to the end of the hall.

"Mom, we're going out for a little while. We'll be back later."

There was no way to reason with or cajole her. No matter how much I wished she could understand and accept the move, I knew she could not.

Vera showed us to the door and opened it, causing an alarm to go off. She quickly showed us how to punch in the code to stop the sound, and we slipped out the door. Through the small window in the door, we could see Vera take Mother gently by the hand and lead her toward the nursing station. The distraction was long enough. By the time Mother was lucid enough to realize we had left, it wouldn't matter. She would soon slip back into the haze of dementia, unaware of our absence.

143

Later that day, Michele and I returned to see her. I brought some movie musical videos from my collection.

"Vera, do you think the ladies might enjoy a musical?"

"It's an excellent idea. We'll play one straight away, after dinner!"

"I thought it might provide distraction and give you a break." Vera loved the MGM musicals, being part of a generation who remembered the likes of Gene Kelly and Fred Astaire.

"Thank you, Chris, we'll look forward to it."

After dinner, the women gathered around a TV set and Vera put *Singing in the Rain* in the VCR. The response from the residents appeared to be very positive. Most of the women sat quietly and watched the film. Mother joined the others and appeared to be content, enjoying the dancing. Michele and I were ready to make our exit.

Unlike a few short hours before, when it had been a wrenching experience to leave Mother, this time we left unobtrusively, or so we thought. As the door opened, the alarm went off. Unlike the first time, this time I was prepared to punch in the code. The shattering noise ceased. Then I understood: There was no quiet way to exit the floor because the alarm always sounded when the door was opened. Without this alarm system in place, the residents might wander away, putting themselves in potential danger. So much for subtle leave-taking, I thought to myself.

After I had moved Mother into Field Hall, I held a sale of her belongings and furnishings at the apartment. She only needed some clothes, toiletries, and a few favorite pictures and stuffed toys that I brought for her. Joyce needed a living room set so that went to her. A friend at my office bought Mother's bedroom set and china. Miscellaneous persons purchased the other pieces of furniture. Michele and I kept a few sentimental items for ourselves. I gave some odds and ends to family and close friends. The remainder went to Goodwill.

144

As I began my new role as a visiting family member, I learned that it was challenging going to and from Mother's ... home. I looked forward to seeing her, but each time I had to leave, I felt sad as I fumbled my way through my exit. Even though I knew that it was necessary and appropriate that Mother was housed in a secure residence, I still felt pangs of guilt at leaving her there and returning to the outside world without her.

When I was ready to leave after a visit, I asked one of the nurses to distract her long enough for me to slip through the door. I couldn't bear to see the look in her eyes when I was departing. She reminded me of a little kid being left at the babysitter for the first time. How could I explain what was happening in a way she would understand?

The staff was at hand to assist Mother through the day and night. They were specialists who knew what to expect as the disease continued its heinous course. Always prepared for the unexpected, the staff knew how to distract, juggle, and respond as various behaviors surfaced.

Administering medications, grooming, helping residents to the bathroom, dressing and interacting with them were just a few of the staff's responsibilities. They held vigil with the dying, comforted family members and counseled visiting physicians.

Leslie, Vera and others assisted Mother with meals, bathing, dressing, and engaging her when she became restless and anxious. These angels provided care when she could no longer do anything for herself. Mother was becoming more and more helpless and could not survive without constant care and maintenance.

I learned to take one day at a time. When I came to visit, she always brightened, smiled and reached for me as I came through the door. I would bring flowers and other treats like her favorite butterscotch candy, made by the English confectioners, Callard and Bowser that would melt in the mouth. Mother, in the past, could finish a whole package of eight pieces in one sitting. I offered her a piece, which I unwrapped and placed in her mouth. She began to choke. She must have forgotten what it was and what to do with. I slapped her on the back and she coughed it up, but after that I stopped bringing her hard candy.

In the beginning I visited frequently, four or five times a week including weekends. During those visits we danced together like an old Vaudeville team. I began by taking her arm and leading her down the hall. Showing Mother a series of steps to a four-four count, she would follow me and repeat the simple pattern with a pivot following. Dancing was what she loved most, and she had retained a sense of music and a basic execution of simple steps.

Down the hall we'd dance, turning and moving to my vocal accompaniment. I laughed at the memory of all the times over the years I had performed for her at home.

As a child, I pretended to be Fred Astaire, improvising props to represent the familiar hat and cane that was his trademark. I found a yardstick in our closet and a convenient chapeau although it was never a top hat in the MGM musical tradition.

Usually I found a knitted cap more suited for a Minnesota blizzard, but it didn't matter; Mother went along with the charade. I was seven years old when she inquired what the yardstick was for. I waved it at her in a precise manner, executed a turn, and quickly responded, "Silly old bean, can't you see that this is my cane?" She laughed and applauded my number with a beaming smile.

I shopped for Mother every few months, replacing worn clothing. Her clothing, made from easy-care fabrics, had to survive dozens of launderings. Her altered physical and mental condition dictated practical clothing, easily put on and removed.

Mother was still animated and energetic when she was having a good day. At this point, she was still responding in sentences but they were simple. I could always spot her in the crowd or see her coming down the corridor to greet me in her bright yellow sweats. I would run to her side like a lost puppy, and she would hug me. I returned her embrace with great enthusiasm. The affection that passed between us had not diminished.

Hi, Mom!"

Wearing a smile that mimicked a happy face decal, she returned an enthusiastic, "Hi, Dear!" She held tightly onto my hand like a little kid being led across a busy street.

"I've missed you, Mom!" My heart would open, and sometimes my eyes would fill with tears of joy, seeing her at that moment.

"Me, too!"

After Mother had been in her new home for a couple of weeks, I started to take her outside so that she could enjoy the fresh air and warmth of August. A typical outing was a drive to Lake Harriet, her favorite since childhood.

Each time we arrived, Mother would marvel at the beauty of her lake. Her eyes would widen as she gazed at the azure blue water. Gentle waves nudged sailboats moored a few feet away from the shore. They bobbed playfully up and down. She loved the richness of late summer, the sun playing off of the greenery accenting the lake's lush shoreline, the beautiful trees perfect for climbing like those in the yard she had climbed so long ago.

Sometimes we would walk slowly around the entire lake. Other times we would walk part of the way and then sit enjoying a box of what Mother referred to as "Lake Harriet popcorn."

Her favorite treat was a cold sweet chocolate or strawberry ice cream cone. She was like a puppy catching the drips of ice cream as they melted slowly off the top of the cone and dripped down the sides. Mother tired quickly and I would take her back to Field Hall exhausted but content.

Our roles had reversed. She was growing more like a child every day and I had become the protective and attentive parent. It was an odd feeling. Now her cognitive ability was non-existent. Her short-term memory was gone. Even her long-term memory was slipping away. I had to let go of the mother I had known and try to accept her transformation.

The Child 20

Now that Mother had become child-like, thoughts of her permeated my days and tugged at my emotions. Standing next to her, I was looking down at the fragile and slender woman beside me, clinging to my arm for support.

As an inquisitive five-year-old I remember looking up at her, my eyes wide with curiosity. "Mommy, what's it like to be tall?" Though she was of average height at five-foot four inches, to me she was a giant. Mother peered down at me and smiled, "You'll know someday, Christine."

An endearing quality in Mother was her delightful storytelling ability. Characters in books came alive and jumped off the page. She encouraged me to join her. I listened and responded for hours on end.

Tales of Uncle Remus was a favorite book of mine. She would become the voice and persona of Brer Bear, Fox, and Rabbit. She would tell me stories on a bus traveling downtown, on a grassy knoll by Lake of the Isles, or in the evening on my bed. Spellbound and hanging on every word, I begged Mother to continue reading even as she became bleary-eyed and eager for a break.

The summer I turned six, we were invited to Boston. We were going to visit Uncle Paul, Aunt Margaret, my cousin Andrea and Paul's in-laws. It was a long trip by train, so she brought along the Uncle Remus book. She read the same stories over and over, until she was hoarse.

As the train wound its way through rural land and cityscapes, I was content, mesmerized by her voice. I listened to the adventures of Brer Rabbit as he outwitted the big, clumsy Brer Bear and the devious, foolish Brer Fox. These travel companions entertained me all the way to Massachusetts.

Back in the mid-40s, passengers paid extra to acquire sleeping berths, preferable to sitting up all night in coach class. Cars known as sleepers held double-decker tiers of small, tented cubicles called berths lining either side of the narrow aisles of the train.

It was fun to get ready for bed, knowing that I could climb into the upper berth and snuggle down under the covers. Mother tucked me in and patiently read to me until I was ready for sleep. It was soothing to hear the train whistle and the clang of the gate at the train crossings along the way. When I could no longer keep my eyes open she closed the book and kissed me goodnight. I fell asleep to the rhythmic, gentle sway of the train.

My other favorite books were A. A. Milne's *Winnie the Pooh*, and *The House at Pooh Corner*. I never grew tired of the adventures of Pooh and all his companions including the irrepressible Tiger. Mother would create tunes to the words of the characters to enhance each adventure. She often said she enjoyed the tales as much as I did. As she turned pages, she laughed loudly, and her enthusiasm was infectious.

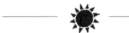

I thought Mother might once again enjoy the stories. I would read to Mother, hoping to jog her memory with the delightful characters she had once loved.

I stopped to purchase the books on my way to visit Mother. I found her by the nurse's station. She enjoyed the attention from the staff aides who were getting to know and like her.

I reached in my purse and showed Mother what I had brought. She looked quizzical until I said, "Pooh Bear." Smiling, she reached up, threw her arms around my neck and followed me down the hall to her room. With her typical enthusiasm, she giggled and smiled as we passed a few wandering but otherwise placid residents. She never noticed them.

I sat on the edge of her bed and she sat down beside me. She cuddled up and listened intently to every word, fully attentive and happy. I remembered the tunes she had sung to me so long ago, and so I sang to her as I read the stories from my childhood. I didn't know if the stories were getting through to the part of her mind holding distant memories or if she was just entertained by the sounds I created.

I realized as I was reading to her, how important it was for me to accept the role of parent with her. Reading aloud was my way of trying to stay in touch with that part of her long-term memory that included my childhood.

Even through my pain, a curious and peaceful feeling came over me. Quietly putting the book aside, I hugged her. Warm tears slowly ran down my cheek. She gave me a shrug and a little sigh. It was time to go for the day. Mother got up with me and I resisted explaining my exit.

Following me to the end of the corridor, she looked at me with an expression that seemed to ask, "Chris, where am I?" She seemed to want to go home, or perhaps that's what I wanted. I'm not sure what she really felt or understood. I punched the security code on the door and slipped out as quickly as I could.

Furtively looking back through the window on the heavy door, I saw a fearful, puzzled, and wide-eyed expression on her face. I hurried away.

A day or two would pass between my visits to the care center. At first, each time I visited, my heart felt heavy with guilt and sadness at having placed her there, away from the world. The feeling would pass as soon as I spotted my sprite of a mother. We would hug and my mood would lift, carried away by our laughter.

I remember a conversation I had with Michele one afternoon when Mother was still living at home.

"Do you know what will be the hardest day of my life?" I waited.

"When Grandma dies?" Michele was direct, which I appreciated in spite of my pain.

"No, it will be when I place her in a nursing home."

"Really, Mom?" My daughter looked at me concerned.

"I'm not sure I can do it." I had been in a state of despair that day and needed to express it. I also knew it was the only choice I could have made.

As time went on, I devised another way to communicate with Mother—through the use of puppets. I would find one I liked and buy it until I had acquired a small collection. The puppets were easy to animate while I created voices and personalities for each.

First there was Leroy, a mangy lion, who was bossy with Mother and tickled her mercilessly.

Next came Big Bird from *Sesame Street*. He was dressed as a bandleader complete with hat and plume, and he held an attached soft fabric bugle. When I pressed it, tiny strains of "Reveille" would play.

My favorite was a gift from Michele to Mother. Super Grover, also a character from *Sesame Street*, arrived complete with a hot pink cape and a big soft bulbous nose to match. I would make him swoop around the room to rescue Mother from imaginary villains.

She would laugh when the puppets sang to her and soon other residents would stop at the door and watch my Henson-like antics. When I finished I would put the puppets all around her bed and silently acknowledge my gratitude for years of training in the theatre and my subsequent life of performing. The puppets were our connection, a link. I was fighting to hang on to any shred of memory she might have. Her responses to me were becoming fewer; her distant memory bank was emptying.

I would try to visit at mealtime so that I could help Mother eat. Her responses to food were slower and more awkward than they had been a few months earlier. She played with her food, moving it around the plate and not eating. At those moments I would pick up the fork and play the game we all remember as toddlers. The morsel of food became the object going into the cave. Mother would cooperate especially if she had become frustrated trying to handle her food. Jell-O and noodles were a challenge and usually ended up in her lap or mine.

She had trouble chewing her food because of her diseased teeth. A few months before she had been diagnosed with degenerative gum disease. At that time we decided to hold off until she could receive full-time professional care while she was recovering from the extractions.

Our dentist Kordie Reinhold suggested oral surgeon Rhonda Altom to perform the procedure. We went through the motions of having her fitted for a denture, had it made, and scheduled the surgery. The surgeon would place the denture in Mother's mouth immediately after the extractions. I was not looking forward to the procedure, knowing that Mother would not understand what was going on, however, the time had come. All Mother's teeth would be removed.

On the day of her outpatient surgery at a local hospital, I drove and Michele accompanied us. Dr. Altom was one of the first women in the state of Minnesota to practice oral surgery. I asked her how periodontal disease starts. She explained that in Mother's case, it could have developed over a period of years, perhaps twenty or more. Mother's earlier smoking and drinking were a big factor in the development of her gum disease. Then she explained the procedure and prepped Mother, and Michele and I went to the waiting area.

During the two-hour surgery, we read magazines, people-watched and together recalled happier days when Mother and Eddie were at the top of their game. A young woman interrupted to inform us that Mother was in the recovery room and could be taken home.

I was not prepared for what I saw when I went to get her. Mother was seated high in what looked like a giant barber chair, dressed in her street clothes. Her legs were straight out in front of her. The denture in her mouth looked like it had been jammed in, forcing a ghoulish grin. Trying to smile bravely when she saw us walking toward her, tears streamed down her face. She must have been experiencing intense pain as the anesthetic wore off.

A nurse practitioner, assisting Dr. Altom handed us pain medication, a list of post surgical instructions and best wishes, adding, "Your mother was a wonderful patient." We helped Mother out of the chair and slowly walked her to the car.

I gently put Mother in the front passenger seat, hooked her seatbelt and tried to avoid bumps in the road during the trip back to Ebenezer. I didn't want to cause any unnecessary, added discomfort. Michele held Mother's hand.

At Field Hall Vera took over and assured us that she and the aides would do everything they could to make Mother's recuperation as comfortable as possible. She gave Mother her medication, and we looked over the post-operative instructions together. The staff was to keep her as quiet as possible during her recovery.

"Chris, she will be confused and in some pain between pain dosages, but your mother will go in and out of awareness and it may not be as tough this way."

"I feel sick leaving her like this, Vera, but I have to get back to work."

"Don't worry. Hels will receive good care. She'll be under the constant surveillance of the staff."

Mother must have felt odd having that appliance in her mouth since she could not understand its use. When asked how it felt her reply was simple:

"It feels big in there!"

I tried to comprehend what she meant. "Big in where, Mom?"

She pointed to her mouth and opened it wide. "In here."

The denture lasted only a week. When she couldn't stand the hardware another minute she pulled the bottom half out, wrapped it in a napkin and placed the wad on her meal tray. When the staff discovered the denture missing, they realized it had been accidentally disposed of. Trying to eat with the remaining part of the denture in her mouth confused her more, so we removed the other half. Mother's gums hardened and she learned to eat without teeth. The nurses were not surprised, but it amazed me!

She was placed on what the staff referred to as a "mechanical soft diet" and enjoyed eating for the first time since she had moved to Field Hall. All her life she had had a dread of gaining a single pound and had been very disciplined in her eating habits. Years earlier, Mother had insisted that she was a person who "eats to live, not lives to eat." Suddenly she was gobbling everything placed in front of her.

I had never seen Mother eat with such enthusiasm. Thinking back over all the years that she had been frantic and fanatical about not gaining weight, it was humorous to watch her new approach to food. Obesity was something Mother abhorred in others including her mother Christina who had been overweight all of Mother's life.

Mysteriously, she appeared to be enduring all the changes so gracefully, calmly and with so much dignity. I marveled at her serenity and docile repose.

At the same time I was chafing and mourning. Each week brought changes that left less of her. The disease was winning.

The Toddler   21

I n the beginning of this journey, it was hard to imagine that Mother would become someone I didn't know. At each level, the change in her was subtle, a skill or memory present one day and then so obviously missing the next. Tucked away was my hope that Mother would stay put. I also prayed she would not experience any sudden transformations or endure terrifying changes.

The disease was also ravaging Mother physically. Comparing a photo taken at a family wedding in September of 1991 to one taken during her second month of residency in August of 1992, I could see a dire change. The disease was aging her quickly, as though on a speeded up film.

Mother could not bathe, brush her teeth, comb her hair, dress, eat or go to the bathroom without assistance. She had become completely incontinent. She would look anxious and take my hand if she had to go to the bathroom. I understood her need by her agitation. At other times, a staff member would remind me that it was time for a bathroom visit. We established a schedule of bathroom visits. If she missed having a bowel movement for a few days, the staff would give her a suppository.

I remember the first time I took Mother to the bathroom at Field Hall. She was wearing a pad. The staff did not refer to this preventative measure as a diaper. All I could think of was my own infancy when Mother changed my diapers. Now the scenario was reversed except Mother wasn't an infant but a grown woman needing assistance. At first, I found it simply too much to handle emotionally. I felt it was beneath Mother's dignity and mine, yet I had no choice but to assist her.

I would turn Mother around in front of the commode, pull down her sweats and underpants, seat her and wait for her to have a bowel movement. When she succeeded, I would help her up to her feet, wipe her, and flush the toilet. I would then pull her clothing back up, turn her to face the basin and run the water, carefully wetting her hands and applying the soap. Once her hands were washed, I dried them with a paper towel, and we would exit the bathroom. It was obvious that Mother had turned into a pre-schooler, needing help like this. The experience was humbling.

Mother was not able to eat without assistance. A staff member or I sat next to her at a table with three other residents. The consistency of having the same three familiar faces at every meal reassured her.

Tying a bib around her neck, I would talk to her as I fed her, describing what she had on her tray. "Oh, look Mother, look at all of this good stuff! Now we're going to start with the turkey, and then you can try some mashed potatoes and gravy.

"Green beans? Look! You love green beans. Yummy!"

She seemed happy at mealtimes especially when she saw me walk into the dining area. Mother attempted to talk to me. Even though her sounds were barely audible, I was pleased that she was trying to communicate. I believe she knew what she wanted to say, but no longer had the tools to make it happen.

She continued to enjoy her food. I would refer to it as "mystery food." Even some of the aides weren't sure it was. Her food arrived looking like mush. The fruits and vegetables were colorful, resembling baby food but lacking aroma, texture or flavor! The meat and potatoes were beige and white sludge on a plate. Much conjecture and some hilarity at times accompanied the aides and my attempts to guess the identity of this institutional cuisine.

As residents deteriorated they exhibited odder behavior, making mealtimes more challenging. Mother would become concerned, shaking her head slightly or muttering under her breath when individuals would act out their frustrations. It was not unusual to hear residents yelling obscenities. They threw objects at no one in particular, and some stomped the floor or pounded the table. Outbursts would go unnoticed by those at later stages of deterioration. The more lucid individuals, still having their social sensibilities intact, called attention to their unruly neighbors.

"Hey, tell her to shut up!" One resident was noticeably upset, tugging at an aide's sleeve.

The aide looked up, trying to locate the source of the complaint. "Who do you mean, Agnes?"

"That one over there!"

"Now Agnes, it's ok. She'll quiet down," the aide said, trying to placate her.

"No she won't. Shut up, you!" In this case, an aide removed the disruptive resident from the table and fed her in her room.

Alzheimer's is an isolating disease. People stricken lose track of where they are. I referred to it as "haze." One minute Mother would be involved with her surroundings, and the next moment she was silent and staring blankly into space. It was as though she were in a vacuum or a bubble looking out at the world.

She was watching somewhere in the Universe, and yet she was entirely alone. Activity swirled around her but she was stuck, unable to relate to or understand what was happening. This woman couldn't be Mother. It wasn't possible. This little lady was docile and silent, not feisty and independent.

As far back as I could remember, Mother had stood up for what she believed in, was strong in her opinions and even more determined in her actions. If anyone had been unfair to me, Mother was always in my corner.

When I turned seven, we moved to Hopkins, a small community west of Minneapolis. Back in the 40s, it was highly unusual to be divorced, and Mother was a career woman and a single mother. She stood out as an oddity in our neighborhood. Certain individuals of the church we attended shunned us.

One day following school, our pastor's daughter Elizabeth, who lived only two houses away from us, invited me over to play. I loved to play with dolls, and she had a whole room full. We were playing with her dollhouse, moving the miniature furniture around, when she looked up at me with a very serious expression on her face.

"Do you know what?" I leaned in, expecting to hear something fascinating.

"No, what? Elizabeth looked around to see if anyone was within earshot and continued.

"I have a secret to tell you, Christine!"

"What is it?" My curiosity was getting the best of me and I couldn't wait to hear what she had to say.

"Your mother's divorced, Christine, and God is going to punish her. Do you want to know how?" Elizabeth was taunting me, laying out the bait. Worried but not wanting to show my concern, I took the hook.

"How?"

"She'll go to hell and burn, that's what!"

I couldn't believe what I was hearing. Tears filled my eyes and I immediately got up and excused myself, running from the house as fast as I could. By the time Mother came home from work, I was inconsolable. Through wrenching sobs, I tried to explain to Mother what our pastor's daughter had said.

As Mother listened, her ire grew. She grabbed me by the hand and headed to Pastor Stohl's house, still wearing the hat and gloves she'd worn to work that morning. Up the front walk and around to the side entrance we marched. Mother beat on the door until the pastor's sister finally responded. A screen door separated us.

"I have something I wish to say to the pastor. Is he home?" Elizabeth's aunt wore a tight expression. In my young mind she was prissy and mean.

She responded with a sanctimonious lilt in her voice, "Why yes he is, but he is not to be disturbed at the moment." Mother persisted, refusing to budge from the doorstep.

"Tell Pastor Stohl that Helen Winter is here and that it is important." The maiden aunt stood her ground and in a haughty voice replied, "I told you, he is not to be disturbed."

I remember Mother trying to keep the lid on that afternoon. She tried to explain to the woman what I had told her. Not only was Mother not allowed to see the pastor, his sister refused to believe that her niece was capable of such a vicious remark and promptly slammed the door on us.

Mother was not about to let the incident pass. A week later, following the church service, she caught up to Pastor Stohl and confronted him as he was leaving the church. She demanded he explain his daughter's behavior. He could not look my mother in the eyes as he mumbled an apology for his daughter's inconsiderate remarks. Mother's honesty and directness had disarmed him, and he took the heat like a gentleman, pastor and a whipped puppy.

I stopped playing with Elizabeth and her pals and found other more accepting playmates.

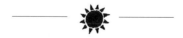

Mother had always looked directly into the eyes of anyone she communicated with. She had taught me that could get and hold anyone's attention. Even as she struggled in the earlier stages of her disease, Mother tried to continue to make direct eye contact. She would focus on me and listen as I spoke to her. I believe that long afterward she had moments when she understood me but could not form a response.

I thought back to the decision I had made in the fall of 1991 when Mother was first diagnosed with Alzheimer's. I called everyone in our family to inform them of her condition. I got a potpourri of responses.

"Alzheimer's, what's that?"

"You've got to be kidding, are you sure?"

"Not Aunt Helen!"

Some of our relatives were casual, not knowing how to respond. A few were distressed. In some cases, I was met with silence. I even heard some skepticism and denial. I'm sure some thought, "That doesn't run in our family, does it?" and "Does that mean I'm susceptible?"

During Mother's first months at Ebenezer, I had still attempted to take her on outings, especially to family functions. These experiences were disappointing for me and stressful for others observing her. Removing her from and then returning her to Ebenezer became traumatic, and I had to suggest that the family visit her there.

Occasionally friends such as Joyce Fowler, her former neighbor, and Martha Schaefer, a friend from her Chowen Avenue years, would visit.

Joel Thom had moved to Florida and wasn't in town often. On one occasion, he visited Mother. I believe he was shocked by her appearance, though he never let on. The first fall of Mother's residency, my friend, Brooke Roma from New York, came to visit. She wanted to see Mother and I brought her to Ebenezer.

Both Joel and Brooke were friends of long standing but Mother had difficulty remembering who they were. This understandably caused them some consternation, but they tried to engage her anyway. It was the only time either of them saw Mother in that condition.

The second month of her residency, my cousin Paul Winter, his wife Pat and their son Paul John came to the Twin Cities to visit. Paul John had never met his Minnesota cousins, so it was an excellent opportunity for the family to get together. My cousin Paul adored his aunt Helen, and naturally wanted to see her.

When Paul arrived at Ebenezer with his family, Mother appeared to recognize him and was also delighted to see Pat and Paul John. They were gracious, kind and happy to see her after so many years, and the attention pleased her.

At my request, Paul and Pat, former opera singers, agreed to entertain the residents. Their glorious voices sang out acapella and many residents came to the lounge to listen.

Even those who usually stayed in their rooms joined the group gathering. Some stood and others sat, transfixed by the lovely sounds soaring through the halls. Even some of the most agitated and combative residents seemed calmer when they heard these beautiful voices reaching out to them.

As his parents performed, Paul John sat quietly holding Mother's hand. She was smiling and swaying as she listened to her nephew's voice. For a few brief moments, I think she remembered Paul and Pat's singing just as they had sung the night of their wedding in Philadelphia twelve years before. She had attended the ceremony. During the reception, the bride and groom performed a number of duets, much to the delight of their guests.

Mother had always been so proud of Paul's vocal ability and she was happy he had married a singer of his caliber. After the reception, she had commented on the romantic ideal of the bride and groom's voices united in soaring song.

When the mini-concert ended, the residents slowly dispersed and we took Mother back to her room. Paul and his family followed close behind, observing the activities going on as the staff prepared for dinner. The dinner cart arrived from the kitchen and staff dispersed trays. I chose to have Mother served in her room so we could all sit comfortably and visit during the meal.

Everyone sat or stood as I fed Mother her supper. She was tiring and losing track of what was happening around her. As she finished her food, everyone continued talking. She paid no attention to our conversation, nor did she make any attempt to join in. Mother sat in the middle of our family group and stared blankly ahead.

Paul caught my attention by holding up Mother's hand. Something greasy was oozing out of her clenched fist. I wrenched the item free, discovering that it was the piece of cardboard a pat of butter had been on. The butter had melted, running down her arm.

Although disconcerting to my relatives, such incidents were routine to me. I went to fetch a washcloth from the linen cart, parked outside of her room. After rinsing out the cloth, I returned and made light of the incident by singing and dancing around Mother as I wiped away the grease singing "Hold that butter, hold that butter" instead of "Hold that tiger, hold that tiger!" She giggled as though it were a game. Once the mess was cleaned up, we all continued with our conversation as if it never happened. After a few minutes, it was evident that Mother needed to rest so our relatives excused themselves.

Paul had known his aunt Helen from the time he was a little boy living in Massachusetts and later as a young man growing up in Honolulu. He was eager to see her whenever he was told she was coming for a visit, and the two were inseparable when she arrived.

The whole family had known her as an independent woman and a free spirit, capable of exploring vast beaches on her own for hours on end, or holding her own at a party, introducing herself and then holding court. Now they were seeing her in the grips of a debilitating disease, not capable of making a single decision for herself and totally dependent on others for her very survival.

Though I had discussed her physical and behavioral changes with them when I called long distance prior to their visit, they had not watched the gradual deterioration as I had, but had seen her only at this moment, and it was a shock. This is a natural reaction to the transformation caused by Alzheimer's. Both the physical and mental changes are startling.

Physically, she had shrunk and had become frail and dependent. Mentally, she was confused and rarely aware of her surroundings. It was a sort of ambulatory coma. This was not the scintillating and facile woman my cousin once knew as his aunt. This lady was a stranger, not his father's lively sister. The disease is hard to assimilate or understand in concentrated form.

One of the obvious developments as a result of the progress of the disease is residents get few visitors. The regulars are those who had taken over the supervision of loved ones legally and physically. Adult children or spouses seemed to be the only consistent visitors. When residents lost their ability to communicate it made visiting awkward. Late-stage residents receive no visitors. Like pariahs, they were left to live out their last years ignored or forgotten.

We become witnesses to life slipping away; it is a frightening reminder of our own fragile mortality. Even the toughest and most steadfast individual buckles under the pressure of the changes experienced as the disease moves forward holding a loved one in its relentless and unforgiving grip.

The Infant 22

C ertain days had been special to Mother. Birthdays, Thanksgiving and especially Christmas were her favorites. The first year Mother was at Ebenezer, we celebrated them all together. At that time, she was still cognizant that something special was going on.

By Christmas morning, Mother had been a resident for four months. I had spent a lot of time wrapping presents for her, using colorful gift-wrap and ribbon adding big red and green bows. All the gifts I selected were colorful clothing. Anything else would have been pointless and impractical.

I placed the brightly wrapped gifts on her bed, and when she saw them she seemed puzzled. I handed her a package and indicated she open it. She sat still holding it, unable to proceed. I slowly opened each gift, adding a running narrative just as I always had. Sometimes this kept her slightly interested, and at other moments, she was totally indifferent.

She looked at each item and touched it briefly but never smiled or expressed pleasure. This was a far cry from the days when Mother acknowledged presents by jumping up and down with delight, squealing and prancing around the room.

After the ritualized gift-giving, I helped Mother try on her new clothes. She appeared to enjoy the activity more than the clothes.

As time passed I still attempted to celebrate the holidays. The Ebenezer staff always tried to create a holiday environment. I would join Mother for dinner, ordering a tray in advance.

I would come early and dress her in a special velour outfit of pants and a matching top that was dressier than her pedestrian sweats. Her clothes size hadn't changed, but she seemed more fragile and I had to help her gently into her clothes. She liked the attention.

Having gotten her ready, I would escort her to the dining hall and seat her in her assigned chair. She was still very ambulatory and enjoyed strolling, her arm hooked to mine. In spite of the changes, she still had a little swagger in her walk.

On Thanksgiving staff dieticians would attempt to create the traditional holiday meal. Mother's food looked as though someone had run the entire dinner through a blender. In my mind it was the same bill of fare, the same sludge served any day.

While Mother's meal wasn't very appealing in appearance or to my taste buds, Mother enjoyed every morsel. Her enthusiasm for food never faltered as I continued to feed her. Because she ate with such pleasure and speed, I barely had time to get the spoon up to her mouth. Missed morsels landed on her chin or her bib.

The dining room décor was always in keeping with a specific holiday. The staff took special pains to provide holiday table decorations too. The ladies would arrive in their special holiday outfits. The staff assisting them wore special colors to match. Place cards marked each resident's spot at the table. The staff put an Easter Bunny, a pilgrim or Santa Claus at the center of each table, depending on the season.

A makeshift chapel for interdenominational church services every Sunday and during holidays was created by arranging rows of folding chairs and placing a lectern and a piano at the front of the room. Some residents attended with family members and staff escorted individuals in wheel chairs or walkers.

Occasionally I would attend the services with Mother and as usual, she seemed to enjoy the activity. She mumbled and pointed, trying to convey her pleasure. She was absorbed and happy and this put me at ease. I was trying to help her continue her lifetime habits as much as possible, although how aware of my efforts she was, I didn't know.

A good friend John Command stopped by to see Mother the first New Year's Eve of her residency. We had been colleagues for years and he adored Mother. Big Band musicians were performing that afternoon. John insisted on taking Mother upstairs to hear the music.

We found her wandering around in her bright red satin bathrobe. She had forgotten we were coming. Nevertheless, I got her dressed and we went upstairs.

Mother appeared to recognize John and smiled when she saw him. Activity room chairs were set up in rows for residents and their guests. Most of the band members were older, retired musicians and they played the music of Glenn Miller and Benny Goodman. They were not polished but no one seemed to care or notice a sour note or two.

John offered Mother his hand. She followed his lead and soon was shuffling to the beat. Later John told me that while they were dancing, Mother looked up at him and said, "Oh, I know you. You're that great dancer!" Somehow she remembered John dancing in many shows she had seen over the years. Mother appeared to connect with anything to do with dance, and during those moments experienced some memory of it. Already tired after dancing briefly, she wanted to sit down. I sensed it was time for Mother to return to the unit. John and I escorted her back. I was always grateful to John for coming to see her that day.

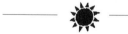

What a contrast this scene was to the picture I held in my mind of my folks dancing years before. Eddie and Mother attended many Shrine functions over the years where Big Bands played and dancing was always the highlight of any party. They both loved jazz and the Dixieland sounds and would often dance the night away. Like a couple of teenagers at a sock hop they didn't know when to stop.

The next day, Eddie could hardly walk. Even though his arthritic knees fought him with each step he took and Mother would be hungover and exhausted, they would regale me with story after story of their previous evening's activities.

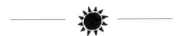

Mother's Day brought more activity to the unit than usual. Many adult children of the residents came to visit. The facility put on a special luncheon and we were all invited to the activity area. I recall bringing Mother a bright summer hat to wear.

Within a few minutes of joining the festivities already in progress, Mother began to fidget and complain. She was clearly not enjoying herself. I had a hunch she saw nothing but old people around her and felt uncomfortable. In a brief moment of lucidity she couldn't equate herself with the elderly women there.

Once again I was forced to let go of my expectations and stop hanging on to what was. Knowing she couldn't experience any of her former pleasures, I knew the best choice was not to force her participation, but I was sad another special day was lost.

Later looking back on that day, I realized that it was a blessing that Mother wasn't really aware of her own aging. She would have despised the way she looked. When she had turned sixty-five, she scorned the opportunities and discounts afforded senior citizens. She refused to have any part of growing old. Now Alzheimer's had speeded up the process and it was out of her hands entirely. The deterioration was more rapid than the normal aging process and mercifully the disease spared her from having to watch it.

One month later in June of 1993, on the first birthday Mother celebrated at Field Hall, I ordered a bunch of balloons for her and had them delivered. Hours later, I dropped by after work to see her and her room was filled with shifting colors and streamers as the balloons floated in a corner. One couldn't help but see them against the stark colorless walls, yet Mother seemed unaware of them. Alzheimer's was gradually erasing all holidays from her memory. After that first year I had to stop celebrating special days with Mother. They were just another exercise in futility.

Holidays and other special days had always been festive and everyone was welcome in Mother and Eddie's home. My cab would pull up in front of the house on Chowen Avenue, which was covered with bright red lights for Christmas, red being Mother's signature color. Huge piles of snow lined the curbs throughout Minneapolis. At times they were so high that from the inside of the taxi I couldn't see over them.

As I stepped out of the cab I could hear music from a loudspeaker mounted over the front door. Sometimes I would hear the mellow voice of Nat King Cole singing "The Christmas Song," and on occasion Bing Crosby's smooth baritone voice would fill the entire neighborhood with "White Christmas." Visible from the front steps, the Christmas tree's bright red lights blinked, beckoning me into the warmth of the house.

Inside Mother, dressed from head to toe in red, threw her arms around me in an enormous hug.

Behind her Eddie stood with a big grin on his face waiting his turn. He wore a bright red bow tie and on his sleeves a pair of sequined arm garters sparkled, catching the light. It was impossible to be a Grinch in that house.

The tree was majestic, trimmed with a unique collection of glass ornamental birds as well as Mother's red lights.

Eddie always prepared the other holiday bird, stuffing it with his famous dressing that he started preparing the night before. Those partaking of his secret recipe over the years agreed that he had the best turkey dressing. My parents always welcomed a few additional people having no other place to go. There was always room at the LaCaze table.

Eddie prepared his infamous Stingers after dinner. He used both white and green crème de menthe, and consuming more than one of his drinks left guests indulging in a long winter's nap. He was a congenial host and with Mother at his side he loved to hold court after dinner. Mother's mischievous humor and clever wit sparked any occasion. Everyone who knew my folks loved and respected them.

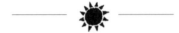

Those Christmases were long gone. Mother sat indifferent and confused, unaware of the passage of time. Gone were the days of her marriage and the fellowship and conviviality of splendid times. She was starting to require constant attention. She was reverting to an infant-like state. She had no awareness of time, place, routine or self. Her abilities, social skills, and values were gone. She was engulfed in non-existence.

Less Is Less

In my former profession as a dancer and choreographer "Less is more" became my credo after working for my late mentor, choreographer and director, Bob Fosse. In time, I applied the phrase to Mother's life.

By her second year at Ebenezer I had stopped wrapping elaborate Christmas presents for her. I began scaling down her possessions. Mother had left most of her personal property behind when she moved there. The stuffed animals and hand puppets that at first sparked her attention had ceased to interest her. Now, just holding her hand and speaking clearly and quietly was enough to elicit a smile. Life was basic.

A formal portrait of Mother and Eddie hung over the head of her bed. Each time I walked into her room and saw that photograph, I was reminded of what her life had been at one time. The two of them had been best friends, partners and soul mates, and the memory of their relationship filled me with both gratitude and sadness. She wasn't even aware of the photograph.

Articles of clothing got lost in the vast laundry system but eventually returned. Toys disappeared from her room. Other residents picked them up as they wandered in and out her room. The toys remaining in her room were now soiled. I decided to take them home to wash. I didn't return them to her room. Instead, I gave them away to friends with young children.

I kept greeting cards taped to the mirror of her bureau, as well as a few snapshots. Mother was unaware of them, but I left them there to add color and interest for visitors. Mother could no longer communicate with them. Her jumble of sounds and words made no sense.

e months passed, I became aware that less was more for unit. It was important to respond moment by moment to events there. Each resident lived in a fixed reality of her own. Everyone else was an observer outside that reality and couldn't know for sure what the individual resident's reality was. It was important to respond to their sounds and gestures not logic. I had no idea what an individual might be thinking, how they perceived me, or if they could think or perceive at all. Their actions and speech patterns were jumbled, and their moods were random and unreadable.

One resident named Pauline loved to stop by Mother's room to visit. She apparently liked me, following me around the unit as I visited with staff and other residents. She was in her mid-eighties and spoke only in grunts. I loved her wide, expressive eyes, much like a toddler's curiously exploring the world around her.

Pauline was always beautifully dressed, usually in a pretty print frock with matching earrings and a necklace. Her hair was done neatly and her demeanor was gentle and sweet. A staff person told me that she had been the daughter of a cattle rancher. As a young girl she had assisted her father, often driving the herd from the open range back to the stock pen at the end of day.

During one of my visits Pauline wandered into Mother's room, and sat down with us on the edge of the bed. She looked lovely, as always.

"Pauline, what beautiful black beads you're wearing." Her gentle demeanor suddenly gave way to a stern look in my direction.

"They're not black, they're blue." She was adamant, and I felt no need to contradict her. I played along, using my improvisation skill.

I ran my hands over them remarking, "Oh, now that I look more carefully, I see that they are blue. Pauline, they're absolutely beautiful blue beads!" She got up and left the room oblivious to my response, but I smiled to myself.

It didn't matter what color the beads were. She was content. I had learned a lesson in accepting the reality of others and not forcing the issue. This helped me deal with Mother as well.

The residents and staff became my extended family. I began to see fewer and fewer visitors on the unit as residents' health declined. When I came for a visit, I often went from room to room to check on favorite individuals. I looked for those who used wheelchairs, stopping to greet them. I spoke their names or sang a few bars of a familiar song. Some would smile. Others sat and stared.

One woman strapped into a wheelchair for her own protection would call out in an agitated voice, "Where is my daughter?" Her eyes would grow steadily wider and more frantic.

"Where is she? When is she coming?" She apparently lived for her daughter's visits.

I would stoop down in front of her, take her hand in mine and speak her name. "I'm sure she is on her way." She'd brighten, and loosen her grip on my hand.

I was humbled watching those with Alzheimer's. It was as if they were living in a vault, locked up tight. You had no possible way of knowing if you had gained access.

From my observations, I guessed that their minds would function for a bit but shut down in an instant. It was like a short circuit, like a light flickering on and off at random and for unpredictable periods of time.

I wonder to this day what Mother felt like going in and out of her haze. I wonder if she had any thoughts or pictures in her head. Behind her eyes I could see an immense effort to communicate, but the words would not come. The connection between ideas and vocal chords failed somewhere in her brain.

After some of these visits I would drive home screaming at the top of my lungs. The frustration and hopelessness of watching Mother's gradual deterioration was often more than I could bear.

It was not fair. My mother did not deserve such a fate and I had no power or control over her destiny. My only power was willingness to let go and accept that there was nothing I could do except to be there for her.

I continued to attend my adult children support group once a month. At each meeting, I would see new faces. I would hear similar stories over and over with a common thread, Alzheimer's. Not only does the illness strip the person of functional and cognitive abilities, the personality changes drastically. Those who had meek and mild personalities might become violent or combative while others who were feisty like Mother had been might become mild and calm.

At this juncture in Mother's residency at Field Hall, she had to move to a total care floor in Luther Hall, located in another wing. Its staff was trained to handle her latest level of decline.

The staff loved caring for Mother. She was cooperative and sweet. Her spirit would break through the wall of dementia and she would laugh. Her laugh was as infectious as ever. It didn't seem to matter what motivated her laugh. Laughter just bubbled up from her toes.

These moments kept me going. Her laughter was an affirmation to me that some part of Mother's old spirit persisted. She was still Helen LaCaze. "Her core is still intact," remarked Jeanne Johnson, a unit nurse on day shift. Her remark brought me great comfort. Jeanne was right. Mother's soul was infinitely alive.

The staff at Luther Hall modeled fortitude and patience watching over those afflicted with dementia. The aides maintained a firm but kindly response with the residents. Aides took enormous verbal abuse.

Occasionally I witnessed a volatile outburst or a barrage of profanity aimed at a nurse or aide. It was ironic to watch some of the largest male aides being targets of such inflammatory language from elderly, frail female residents. At times residents physically assaulted the aides, but that was unusual. Mostly they delivered vile tongue-lashings. The staff monitored combative residents carefully.

I recall one mealtime incident. We were seated at a large round table with other residents. One woman began cursing everyone and throwing food. Utensils followed, and then she topped off her outburst by throwing her dish and plastic cup. She continued to reach for any object she could get her hands on. Mother sighed repeatedly and rolled her eyes.

The noise was loud and disconcerting. Soon others at our table became agitated. One lady began shouting with garbled disdain. Another waved her arms. I was concerned someone might get hurt or become combative too, creating a chain reaction.

As I looked around the dining area for a familiar staff face, I could only catch the eye of a pool worker, a substitute for a regular staff person. The young man was over six feet tall and built like a NFL linebacker. I explained the situation mostly through large gestures. He nodded and in broken English said, "I take care of, Miss." As he reached down to remove the woman in question, she screamed profanities that would have made a deviant blush. He ducked as she swung repeatedly. Many residents overlooked this wild confrontation, but visiting relatives watched with curiosity.

"Unreal. The entire scene is like a bad dream. It's surreal. What a far cry place this is from the world outside," I mumbled under my breath.

Another time I went up to see her in these new surroundings and found her seated next to an aide who was painting her nails. She still recognized me when I appeared. A smile lit up her face.

I hugged her and hung on for a long time, feeling like a little kid not wanting to let go, just as I had when she was leaving for work in the mornings before I started school. I remember standing at the kitchen window watching her as she walked down the alley, taking a short cut to the bus line. When she had disappeared from sight, I felt a twinge of sadness. It was the same now. I wanted her back.

Broken Doll   24

W hen Mother retired at age sixty-five, she had the same fitness
as an active woman of thirty-five. Blessed with good health
all her life, she continued to have incredible energy, enthusiasm
and vitality.

She had followed a regimen of daily exercise that included
biking, swimming and walking. She slept well, maintained sound
eating habits and relaxed either by reading or taking a long walk.

Her yearly exams were always normal, and her doctor's only
advice was, "Wear your seat belt and take calcium supplements."

Being Caucasian, slender and small-boned, Mother fit the
high-risk profile for osteoporosis.

During one of her Hawaiian getaways in the late 80s,
Mother had had an accident. She was walking along the ocean
and tripped in uneven sand. Falling into the surf, she broke her
right wrist. She made light of it. However, in the next few hours,
her pain became more intense and she went to the emergency
room. An x-ray identified the injury as a compound fracture.
Her brother Paul encouraged her to stay in Hawaii longer that
year to recuperate. Mother was delighted to extend her vacation
and heal while enjoying a few more weeks of sunshine. After her
fall she decided to be more careful, admitting she was
"breakable!"

Now, suffering with Alzheimer's, Mother seemed to have lost
all her awareness of hazards. One afternoon, she had wandered
away from the dining room after lunch unnoticed. Sometime later,
a staff worker found her on the floor near her bed. They could not

tell how long she had lain there, unable to move or call for help. They discharged her to the hospital and called me at home.

"Hels has broken her femur and will require surgery. It's been scheduled tomorrow morning at Abbott Hospital."

"I'll meet her there."

I immediately phoned my boss and explained what had happened. In his usual magnanimous fashion he gave me the next day off, wishing my mother well.

The next morning the weather was cold, dreary and sleeting. Wearing a raincoat over a heavy sweater, jeans, tennis shoes and a comfortable hat, I dashed out to my car and drove to the hospital in rain. It fell harder as I pulled into the ramp and parked. I felt comfy dressed as I was, walking through the bleak, damp parking ramp toward the elevator. Downtown Minneapolis was awash with a gray only March in Minnesota can achieve.

Mother's surgery was scheduled for ten o'clock. I signed the necessary paperwork and headed to the cafeteria to get breakfast. I read a magazine I had brought, and then headed back upstairs to the visitor's lounge.

Two hours later I was getting sleepy. I briefly closed my eyes to meditate when I heard, "Miss Winter?"

I looked up into the eyes of a middle-aged gentleman wearing green scrubs. Speaking softly, he said, "Your mother came through the surgery just fine. It was a clean break that will mend well." The cold gray that had colored my morning lifted. Thanking him, I gathered my things and headed up to the recovery area. When I looked in, Mother was fast asleep, so I left.

Later that afternoon, I found Mother lying on her back in bed, staring at the ceiling and jabbering incessantly. She didn't acknowledge my presence as she fidgeted and twisted the sheet. She had no idea where she was and I knew it was pointless to try and explain.

Mother remained in the hospital a few more days. I brought Joyce up to see her. She had settled down and was happy to see friendly faces. She smiled when Joyce spoke to her. Jerry Stamm, another friend from my first support group, stopped by. He adored Mother and was happy to see her. Again she responded with a smile when she saw him.

In a few days she returned home to Ebenezer. The staff was happy to welcome her back.

At first, Mother appeared to be responding to daily physical therapy. The therapist carefully stretched her injured leg. They encouraged her to walk, supported by staff.

She was devoted to the effort and the staff was impressed. Her constructive attitude and progress continued for about ten days.

Then everything changed.

Mother suddenly balked. Agitation replaced her usual sweet and calm demeanor. She cried out when an aide adjusted her position in the wheelchair or placed her in bed. I believe Mother's brain had kicked in, and she realized how completely others were in charge.

On one occasion, a caregiver was taking her to the bathroom and when Mother tried to put weight on the injured leg she refused to budge. It took two aides to lift her to the commode.

It hurt to put weight on her injured leg. She refused to use both legs. In her confusion, she undermined her own healing.

It was difficult to watch Mother's discomfort. I wished that she could comprehend that the staff was trying to help not hurt her, but I knew she couldn't. The unit supervisor agreed that Mother needed to feel comfortable. They stopped pressuring her to move. As a result, she became inactive and lethargic, and began to lose her will.

She was now totally dependent on a wheel chair and bedridden. This was hard for me to accept. For a few weeks, the staff placed Mother in a lounge-type chair that could be moved from her room to the lounge and back again. She couldn't sit upright and sitting reclined looking straight ahead made it hard for her to see or relate to the activity around her, adding to her isolation.

Mother developed a bladder infection during this time. She became weak and unresponsive. The standard medications weren't working.

One of the staff nurses suggested I look into hospice service for Mother. Hospice workers would visit her around the clock and monitor changes as she declined.

In everyone's opinion she was dying. Mother's decline had come on so fast that I was not prepared to let her go. I felt that my Higher Power was acting too quickly. I didn't want her to die. She had been doing so well. This change was too sudden.

Eventually, I came to realize that I had to let go and consciously accept what was.

The hospice workers left me a notebook to read with individual entries made by each worker. This sharing was uplifting and encouraging.

The consensus was that Mother was wonderful to work with even in her present condition. One note read, "Dear Christine: Your mother is a wonderful woman. She smiled at me today when I held her hand." I looked forward to the new entries and notes each time I visited. One of my favorite entries read: "I painted Hels' fingernails today. I used bright pink polish and she really liked that. Your mother is great!" These notations filled me with gratitude.

Once I accepted the fact that Mother might not recover, I began to take care of final details. I created a memorial service that would be a tribute and celebration of her life. I chose participants who readily accepted the roles I suggested. Jimmy Martin, a talented performer and friend, agreed to play the service. With Jimmy's gift for music, I knew that Mother would be pleased. He'd play the songs that had been favorites of hers through the years.

A mix of family and friends would eulogize her. A special photo of Mother would be displayed, showing her warm smile and beautiful, laughing eyes. The service would be held at the chapel at the Cremation Society of Minnesota that was spacious and yet felt intimate. Then I turned the whole thing over to my Higher Power, accepting that this was the best and only choice for me.

To my astonishment and relief, Mother came around. In a matter of weeks, she had overcome the infection that had been keeping her down. She was frail and looked as breakable as a Dresden doll. Her complexion was paste-like and devoid of color. However, she was responsive and was cooperating fully with the staff.

Her appetite returned and it was ferocious. She responded to her caregivers with sounds and her humor was resurfacing. The nurses on both day and night shifts put in a request for Mother to have her own wheelchair. They wheeled her everywhere on the unit. She seemed responsive to everyone.

I tried to limit my visits to the weekends. After a workweek, I needed the relaxed pace of the weekend to put me in the frame of mind to cope with visiting Mother's unit. It was amazing what a full night's sleep would do to rejuvenate tolerance and acceptance. I continued to attend my adult children support group at the Alzheimer's Association once a month too.

My visits became simple. I would arrive at noon rested, alert and responsive to Mother's needs. I was ready for unpredictable interaction with other residents. Pushing her down the halls in her wheelchair, I would talk to her knowing full well she could not understand or reply.

I would occasionally stop and walk around to the front of the chair, making eye contact and greeting her as if I had just arrived:

iom, how are you doing today?" Then I would sing a meuicy of simple tunes. Though she couldn't join me, she would smile when she heard the musical sounds.

The chair ride had replaced our walks and little dance patterns of the first two years. Mother sat still in the chair, a blank expression on her face. Her feet could no longer carry her and her voice was silent.

After fifteen minutes, I would wheel Mother to her room. Parking her wheelchair by the bed, I made sure to lock the large gray wheels in place. Sitting on the bed facing her, I would begin an upbeat one-sided conversation. I tried to demonstrate the gist of the words by drawing pictures in the air.

I'd hold both of her hands, and try to make eye contact with her. She would stare back at me. When I was leaving for the day, I would hug Mother, saying, "I love you." I would reassure her I'd return. The words were meaningless. I would leave her sitting in her wheelchair, staring straight ahead. My leave-taking would go unnoticed. I would ride down in the elevator alone exiting the lobby past the receptionist desk and out the double automatic doors. Walking down the parking lot, I sometimes found tears running down my face. My mind engulfed in reverie, I would cry all the way home.

Working at Nemer, Fieger and Associates was a helpful distraction at this stage of Mother's disease. Being the company receptionist, I was communicating with people all day either on the phone or at the front desk. I enjoyed the interaction with clients, delivery personnel and employees of the company. I was center stage, administering all the information coming and going out of the office. The job gave me the opportunity to use my communication skills and theatre training. One of my friends at the company even referred to my job function as "working the room."

I cannot stress enough the importance of keeping in touch with friends as you travel down the Alzheimer's road. They provide distraction, support, and warm fuzzies, and they allow you to step away from the disease for a while. Sometimes seeing a familiar face or receiving a warm hug was enough to dispel the thicket of despair that surrounded me at times.

Spending time with my daughter was important too. After Mother first went into the nursing home, Michele and I took a long weekend and drove to the Black Hills. It felt good to be away and to talk about something other than Mother's illness.

We took a few other trips during the years Mother resided at Ebenezer. We traveled to San Francisco, New York City, the Catskills in upstate New York and to picturesque parts of Minnesota. The change of scene put us back in touch with the outside world apart from the insular care facility. We also went to movies and sometimes to a concert or play.

We each find our own path to peace of mind. I had been involved with Siddha Yoga for ten years. It is an eastern philosophy based in Kashmir Shaivism. My involvement continued throughout Mother's illness. The meditation practice helped me to keep in touch with that part of myself that is a source of peace and serenity. When pressures built up, an evening of chanting, meditation and fellowship brought me in touch with my inner spirit.

Sometimes I would stop at Lake Harriet. I'd reflect on the times when I used to walk the lakes with Mother chatting, philosophizing, and solving the world's problems—at least in our own minds and in our conversation. It was helpful, during low moments, to remember the past and how good it all was. By the time I had completed the three miles around the lake, my burden would have lifted and life looked better again. Being alone gave me the solitude I needed, and the physical exercise relieved my body of stress and fatigue.

So much was gone. Those once active legs, belonging to the tomboy, Helen Jane Winter, had become withered and still. They rested precariously on the lip of a wheelchair. Her feet turned in, pigeon-toed, and wore practical slippers. The eyes that once reflected wonder had become fixed in a blank stare.

Her special spirit had been stilled and the world that held such joy for her had disappeared. I suspect her suffering and terror had gradually ceased. Life was the moment. She had no future plans. She had no memories of who she was. I wondered what was going on in her mind.

What were sounds like? What did they mean to her? Were they just gibberish to her as her mutterings were to me? Did she understand hunger or recognize the color of her robe? What was her haze like? Did the broadest sensations give a sense of pleasure or were they unpleasant intrusions? Was Mother in a waking coma? Suspended animation? I shuddered in imagining the answers.

I longed for one more view of the effervescent, dynamic, and spirited woman who had been the toast of so many parties. I heard myself saying quietly to myself, "Oh please God, just one more look at that fabulous woman in red!"

Then I looked around and saw where I was. The youthful, carefree Helen LaCaze had vanished and I was walking down the corridor of a hallway leading to a security-coded protective door. I stepped through into another world, the heavy door closing loudly behind me.

A Different Holiday   25

I nevitably Christmas came around again. With Mother's growing impairment and subsequent inability to participate, I had to forego celebrating with her in the present and spent more time remembering how we'd celebrated in the past.

When I was a child, we always had a Christmas tree, fully decorated with colorful glass ornaments, multi-colored lights and silver tinsel that shimmered from the top of the tree to the bottom branches. I loved the music and the abundant camaraderie associated with the Yule season. Our immediate family was small and most of our relatives were spread out around the country. However, Mother's older brother Vernon, his wife Frances and their kids, Jeff, Greg and Lucinda Winter remained in Minnesota. They always invited us for holiday dinners.

Whether it was Christmas, Easter, the Fourth of July or Thanksgiving, we went to my uncle Vernon's house to celebrate. My aunt Frances, who was a fabulous cook, would put on a glorious spread, followed by coffee, dessert, and after-dinner conversation. I actually enjoyed helping her clean up. It was a perfect opportunity for my aunt, Mother and I to visit and discuss everything from fashion to theatre, and to exchange all the latest recipes.

Jeff and Greg continued the tradition during their bachelor years. They held the holiday gathering at their duplex by Lake Calhoun in Minneapolis. Vernon and Frances were now living in Grand Rapids, Michigan, but they would fly in twice a year, first for Christmas and then for the Metropolitan Opera in May. Relatives would always gather when they came to town. Everyone would contribute to the assortment of goodies:

homemade pies, vegetarian dishes, savory turkey, slow-cooked on the barbecue with all the trimmings added, and an assortment of fresh salads and appetizers. Everyone enjoyed digging into the delightful buffet.

When Jeff and Greg each got married and started raising families, the invitations continued. And at each gathering the center of all the activity had been their aunt Helen.

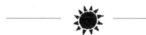

On my seventh Christmas, a school chum told me that there wasn't a Santa Claus. I remember coming home from school heartbroken, and told Mother and Grandma. I had written Santa asking him for a red phonograph and the complete *Nutcracker Suite* since I was a new student of Russian ballet, and loved Tchaikovsky's most popular score. The news about Santa dashed my hopes.

On Christmas Eve since there was no Santa, Mother insisted we open family gifts. When Christmas dawn arrived to my wondering eyes appeared a red phonograph and a square package looking like a record album next to it under the tree. Mother, in her infinite wisdom, had found a way to keep the spirit of Santa Claus alive by holding back the most important presents. I must have played the album all day until I was ordered to bed Christmas night, exhausted but thrilled that Santa hadn't forgotten. Only when I was older did I fully understand and appreciate my mother's actions.

Over the years, we sent Christmas cards and when my grandma Christina was still alive we always had a special dinner served with all the fixings. She would prepare her special sauerkraut and spare ribs with browned potatoes, carrots and pearl onions instead of the more traditional turkey or ham dinner. It was a recipe she carried from the old country and hers was the best.

We eagerly attended Grace Presbyterian Church for its beautiful eleven o'clock candlelight service.

Mother had received her religious education at Grace Church, beginning when the family arrived in Minneapolis from Canada. She had been confirmed there.

I too grew up at Grace, attending confirmation classes and receiving my first communion there. During my high school years, I sang in the church choir, and there was something very special about participating in the holiday services. The minister Morris C. Robinson had been an inspiration to Mother throughout her life and had counseled her through some of her greatest challenges including her divorce. Dr. Robinson was supportive and caring, and he convinced her that she was capable of facing any obstacles in her path.

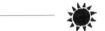

As an adult, I lived far from Minnesota for many years and missed the many special times I might have had with Mother. My career in show business dictated working where the opportunities were professionally and I was only able to visit home twice a year, once at Christmas and once during the summer months. These occasions were celebrations in the truest sense and full of joy. Eddie had come into the picture a year and half before I left for New York, and my new family loved to celebrate together whenever I could return home.

When Eddie passed away at Thanksgiving in 1978, a palpable sadness descended on all of us—especially Mother. She missed him terribly, but would make every effort to feign enthusiasm and keep the festivities going. Yet her spontaneity was missing. I believe part of Mother's spirit died with Eddie.

For the first Christmas without Eddie, I showed up with Michele in tow. It had only been a month and it was a sad time for all of us. Mother put up the tree with the same red lights and glass bird ornaments, but it was clearly not the same.

After that holiday, we all agreed that Mother should come to visit us to get away from the reminders of what had been. Michele and I lived in Detroit, Michigan. I planned a big holiday open house in conjunction with Mother's visits. Camaraderie was in high gear. My Michigan friends always enjoyed Mother and she, them. She was the life of any party and she appeared to be reviving emotionally. It was comforting to us all and we hoped our collective grief would pass.

1995 was another kind of Christmas. I was headed down to Luther Hall alone.

Michele chose not to visit because it made her sad not to be able to communicate with Mother. She had chosen instead to spend the evening with friends. She'd catch up with me later on.

It was twilight when I pulled up in front of Ebenezer Luther Hall located on once-fashionable Park Avenue. The street of old mansions, now converted to businesses or apartments, was mostly silent. The parking lot was empty except for a few staff cars.

Muffled in coat and scarf I walked through the raw winter air, across the cold lot, up the incline to the entrance, and paused for the timed double doors to open.

The evergreen in the lobby was decorated like an impersonal discount store display. Instead of my family greeting me, a receptionist gave me a perfunctory smile and reminded me to sign the visitor's register. The list of signatures was short.

One nurse at the first floor nursing station glanced up, nodding as I walked by. It was eerily quiet without the usual bustle of nurses and aides taking care of residents. The staff must also be home for the holiday, I thought to myself. Mother's floor was also quiet. Another tree stood alone in the common area, blinking garishly, covered in tin foil and cotton snow.

Families who could, brought loved ones home for a few hours, but the majority of residents, unable to leave, remained overseen by a staff of temporary workers.

Not seeing Mother in the common area, I asked for her, but the substitute aides didn't know who she was. They were just filling in because they needed the hours. Ebenezer was just another care facility full of strangers.

I found her sitting in her wheelchair facing the wall in her room. She had been dressed in a faded housecoat with only socks on her feet. Around her neck she wore her glasses on a chain. The incongruity of Mother wearing glasses was obvious; she had no need of them. A pool aide had obviously grabbed the easiest garment to put Mother in instead of some of her more colorful sweats. When I saw her so carelessly dressed my spirit momentarily fell. But when I turned her wheelchair around, I bent down and gave her a bear hug. She was so frail I thought she might break in my arms, but she brightened a bit when she saw me. My spirits lifted. It was difficult to tell if she knew who I was but I guessed that she was happy to see someone, anyone, at this point.

It was getting late for supper. No one from the staff had come to fetch Mother and I assumed she might be hungry, so I wheeled her down the hall to her place at the table where two others already sat.

Once again, the dining room was decorated with Christmas centerpieces at each table and personal name cards marked each resident's seat. The meal was a traditional holiday offering. Mother had her usual plate of soft, blended food, placed in little piles.

I tied a bib on her and sat down to feed her on a stool one of the aides provided. She took each spoonful quickly and ate everything on her plate. I ate my meal, ordered earlier, and though it looked like turkey and the trimmings, I found it bland and boring. With a number of the more alert residents absent it

191

was quiet in the dining area, and most of the other diners sat unaware of their surroundings, being fed by the fill-in staff.

After eating, I pushed Mother's wheelchair down the corridor to a new lounge on a new wing. The large, newly appointed room was more pleasant than the common area. The twilight outside had passed and the windows were dark. Strings of colored lights, mounted on plastic garlands, hung from the ceiling and descended in scallops around the entire room. Another impersonally decorated tree stood in one corner. The lights blinked on and off to a medley of computer-generated Christmas carols. The display seemed garish and glitzy, like a Las Vegas casino but cheaper. I walked around the room inspecting this contrived display while Mother sat silently in her wheelchair. I returned to where she was sitting, pulled over a chair to be close to her and looked around the room once more.

Had it all really come to this? Looking at Mother, I was filled with a lonely melancholy. Suddenly, words began tumbling out, building in intensity and momentum as I let them fly.

"Mom, I miss you so much. I'm not sure what it feels like to be heart-broken, but the way I feel right now must be close to it. I miss everything about you. I miss the old mother: the one who read to me on the train, who showed up at my shows, who was cordial to all my friends, who loved butterscotch, ice cream and nature. I miss your witty sense of humor, your enthusiasm and infectious laughter. But most of all, I miss your common sense, feisty spirit, honesty and wisdom. I miss sharing Christmas with you!"

My heart ached. Reaching over and hugging her to me the floodgates opened. I sobbed and sobbed, holding on to her as she sat completely unresponsive. She never moved.

I felt like I was with a stranger or worse. I was alone. I felt like a little kid who was separated from my only parent. I couldn't find my way back to where she was because she wasn't there anymore. She would never be there again.

Time passed. My tears stopped. I stood and unlocked the large wheels on the chair and we returned to the corridor and down the hall. As I wheeled Mother, I hummed *Santa Claus Is Coming To Town*. My plaintive, less than enthusiastic humming filled the quiet hallway as I wheeled Mother past empty rooms as well as occupied ones where sleeping residents lay oblivious to the eve of Christmas. As I rounded the corner and headed to her room, the last one at the end of the hall, I finished with *Rudolph,The Red-Nosed Reindeer*. I smiled as I remembered the lyrics I learned so long ago in elementary school.

I left her sitting in the wheelchair by her bed. Leaving the quiet floor, I returned to the almost deserted reception area, signed out, returned the visitor badge and wished the receptionist a "Merry Christmas." Walking through the evening darkness to my car, the cold, clean air hit my nostrils and I could clearly see my breath in front of me.

I shivered as I slid into the frosty car, started the engine, turned on the heater and waited a few minutes for it to warm up.

The drive home was sad. Memories returned as I thought about the many Christmases past. I thought about the small white house on Chowen Avenue, trimmed with red shutters. I could visualize the blinking red lights that could be seen all over the neighborhood. I felt the cozy warmth of the fireplace in the living room with Eddie tending it lovingly. I had carefully wrapped the colorful packages under the tree in the privacy of the den. I would warn Mother, Eddie and Michele to stay away until I was finished.

I thought about Michele, the eager little girl who put out a plate of snacks for Santa Claus so he wouldn't starve on his rounds. And I thought about how this evening she had to find solace and distraction with friends because she couldn't bear the sight of her fragile and waning grandma isolated in her haze. Most of all, I thought about my Higher Power sustaining me this Christmas Eve.

Later, I picked up Michele and we attended a late evening service in my neighborhood. Our individual moods blanketed the joyful feelings we had had on so many Christmases past. Everything had changed in our lives because our holidays had revolved around Mother. This Christmas had been about me, about my feelings of loss, rather than about her.

As it turned out, this was the last Christmas Mother and I had together. With each passing week, she was moving closer to oblivion. It was time to update her living will.

Mother's desire had been to have no aggressive medical treatment when she was failing. When possible I had kept her involved in all decisions regarding her future while she was still lucid. She had signed the first draft when she was still living in her apartment.

Recently Kelly Leonard, who was head nurse on the night shift, suggested that I update the document. After thinking it through, I changed her living will to request that she be made comfortable only. This seemed compatible with the spirit of Mother's earlier request. How strange it was to be making this decision marking the end of her life, when the picture in my mind was still the active, carefree, and vibrant woman, Helen LaCaze.

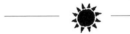

Mother had been like Auntie Mame or the Pied Piper. Everyone loved being around her. Her exuberance was unmatched and she always made each person feel special. Each one of Vernon's kids had stayed at the LaCaze home at one time or another.

Jeff visited often, bringing his buddies by for homemade chocolate chip cookies or Mother's special cake made with rhubarb from her garden.

Greg had hung out with my folks every chance he got, and stayed on weekends when he was home from college. It was

Mother who comforted him and took him to the airport when he left for Vietnam.

Lucinda lived with Mother for a while. They were more like girlfriends than aunt and niece. Mother was like "Dear Abby" as she listened to Lucinda's concerns about her suitors.

Mother was a people person to the core. She always had time to listen and advise. But no matter what personal trials were challenging her, she never let on what they were to others. She never lost her sense of humor or integrity. She was tough, a product of her generation. After all, she and her family had survived the Great Depression and survived it well.

As the months wore on, Mother had fewer visitors. Her brother Paul would call from Hawaii for an update occasionally. Our conversations were consistently the same, with very little variation.

"Christine, this is Uncle Paul."

"Oh, Uncle Paul, it's good to hear from you."

"How's my little sis?"

"She's holding her own. No better, no worse."

He also wrote a letter to me in which he said, "I am enclosing a letter that maybe you can read to Helen. I don't know whether she will understand all of it, maybe some. Chris, your ma is a great gal and I am most happy to have had her all these years as a sister. I love her and only wish that I could do something. I feel so helpless. Please keep me up to date and if I can be helpful, please write me or if time is short please call me and reverse charges. Love, Uncle Paul." As I read his enclosed letter her, containing many reminisces, I was moved by his closure. "Little sister, there are so many memories and I would like to spend time remembering them with you, at your side. You're a wonderful sister and I love you dearly and always will. Paul."

Her other surviving brother Vernon lived in Grand Rapids, Michigan and didn't visit too often. When he was in town visiting his grown children, my cousins and their families, he would stop up to see Mother. The staff would inform me when he had visited though I didn't see him myself.

My cousins Jeff, Greg and Lucinda visited periodically, but they must have found it hard to see their aunt Helen slipping away. She had been a central figure in their lives and now she was mysteriously unaware of them. She was a shell, vacant. No one came to see her.

Those who had known her, had spent time with her, and had trusted her, didn't know the frail lady seized by the disease. The silent, staring woman was too great a contrast to the vivacious Helen LaCaze. Gone were the homemade cookies, rhubarb cake and poetry, the extra bed and the sound advice. Everyone was poorer for the lack of her.

The Silence   26

I guess we all talk to ourselves once in a while. I had all my life. Being an only child I would keep myself busy talking to imaginary playmates, amusing myself for hours. This was an asset when I trained as an actor in New York. Along with my fellow acting students, I'd improvise scenes in which we were required to create spontaneous dialogue.

During the last year of Mother's life, I was grateful for this improvisational skill. I would say things to her hoping for a response but none would come. I would tell her about what I was doing and what was happening in the outside world, and I wondered what, if anything, was getting through. It was a peculiar activity but one that I became good at.

Sometimes Mother would stare blankly, looking nowhere in particular. At other times she would look right through me and I could only imagine what she might or might not understand. She was by now frail and little. She sat slouched in her wheelchair, her hands motionless and her feet still. The chair seemed much too large for her. She sat silent and expressionless, without even the trace of a smile. She seemed totally absent from the spin of outer activity and yet, on a deeper spiritual level, I believe her soul remained present. Mother appeared serene, silent and still.

The regular staff was good about reporting her decline and what changes in her care were needed as she reached a new level of deterioration. They were a wonderful support group for me and I appreciated their insight and experience.

On one occasion, I had wheeled Mother back from the dining room when I spotted Janet Foster of Housekeeping. Janet was always cheerful and was very taken with Mother. She had been attentive to Mother from the moment she was transferred to the fourth floor unit.

I parked Mother by the door of her room and walked a few feet down the hall to chat with Janet for a moment. We had a common interest in cats and would share the latest news about our pets. Our conversation was very animated that afternoon, and as I turned to check on Mother, I was stunned to see her staring at me with a look that seemed to say, "Listen, kid, you came to see me, so come back here!"

I took the cue, excusing myself from Janet, and returning to Mother's chair. Before reaching her I executed a traditional time step, finishing with an upraised, poised arm, the other pointing right at her. In true show biz style I concluded, "Ta Dah!"

She looked at me and with a deep and very audible sigh said, "Oh, Chris!"

I was stunned. My heart leaped and tears came to my eyes. This was the first recognition, the first clear words I had had from Mother in over a year. My little dance step and pose had shaken something loose in her memory bank.

She recognized me—through the most basic of dance steps. Dancing, the one activity she had loved fervently, continued to link us. And, then it was gone. The vacant stare returned. That moment was a special gift, given when I needed it most.

The journey of Alzheimer's is strewn with anger, fear, guilt, helplessness, regret and sadness. This experience also built in me acceptance, patience, resolve, surrender and above all, the will to see it through. My willingness to accept what was left of Mother and cherish that portion had been restored through her awareness of me, if even for a few seconds. The futility of all the times I had visited her without getting a response vanished in a moment. This one moment lit up all the dark months of her passivity.

As time slipped by, fewer visitors came to the unit. And each of my visits became lonelier. Even close relatives gave up communication with their loved ones when they got no overt response to their hopeful prodding. A natural assumption is that when the lights are out no one is home. From Mother's rare response, I knew that's not always true.

The quietness of an Alzheimer's unit can seem eerie as opposed to the normal bustle of activity on other floors where residents are helpless, old, sick and dying but can still communicate. Even the staff seems to move more quietly. There is a palpable stillness, broken once in a while by the outburst of a combative resident, or the repeated crying out of someone muttering nonsensical communications over and over. The whole effect is like watching a motion picture in slow motion with no sound.

I admired the professional caregivers on the dementia units. They were dedicated workers, and they were flexible and responsive to the needs of the residents. The disease causes unpredictable behaviors that are not easy to manage. Each case is different and in Mother's case, she became calm and docile. Mother had seemed to welcome the interaction with the staff in the beginning, though as time went on she could not respond back.

She had become totally dependent on the staff for assistance with all her basic needs and functions and the staff responded to her with devotion and empathy. I used to remark to the staff how easy she was to care for, almost forgetting the nightmare years earlier when she was still living in her own apartment and struggling with uncertainty.

I remembered how she had struggled to remember things during the early onset of the disease. I would think to myself that she should stop fighting the obvious, let go. How ignorant and arrogant of me. I wasn't fighting to hold on to my mind. She was struggling to maintain a hold on reality, and often only more mental chaos was the result. How terrifying it must have been for her.

All of her life Mother's mindset was that she controlled her world. She handled all the departments of her life with dedication, tenacity, and total honesty. She was proactive rather than reactive. In her view, she made things happen. Never one to sit around and cry at her lot, she turned the challenges along the way into opportunities.

When the disease began to rupture her life, she had made the remark that became a clear statement of prophecy: "I can stand anything except to lose my mind." She never expressed in words her terror except for that one time.

She evolved into a dependent child and in time, an infant. This transformation was painful and difficult for me to adjust to, and yet I had accepted the inevitable.

My understanding kept me on my feet as a family caregiver. Without my resignation and surrender, the road would have been paved with even more pain and bitterness. I saw this happen to others when they couldn't accept the disease and refused to face the realities of its progress.

Mother's deterioration had begun in little ways subtle enough to keep me guessing for a year and a half.

In the months she still lived at home, we coped with her growing impairment until we accepted the fact that we couldn't handle the demands of care-giving on a day-to-day basis.

Moving her to a care facility felt as though we were handling a double-edged sword, and no matter how careful we were, we would still get cut. Sometimes Mother's decline stalled for months at a time. Then, as sudden and intimidating as a lightening strike, a drastic change would occur and Michele and I would have to surrender to her further impairment.

A curious aspect of the Alzheimer's journey is that family members and friends observing the stricken person have time to adjust to it. It doesn't occur swiftly, like an accidental death. One has the opportunity to gradually accept it on one's own terms.

When enough losses pile up, our ability to let go becomes honed. It is the kind of experience that tests our mettle, willpower, and tolerance. One discovers his or her strength of character.

A thought that repeated often in my mind was, "No one said it was going to be easy. You do what you have to do."

One of Mother's astute observations on the formation of character had been "Be glad for the lumps. They beat you into some kind of person." They are gifts, oddly enough. They were to me. The disease changed her but it also changed me.

During the course of Mother's disease, I grappled with her decline one level at a time. Temporary let-ups helped me prepare for the next change. These breathers helped me cope, but even so, they didn't prepare me for what lay ahead. I didn't know how difficult the final loss would be.

Time For Goodbye 27

S pring and summer came and went without a drastic change in Mother. It was late fall, 1996. Daylight ended early and the cold was moving in. Time once again to prepare for the inevitable Minnesota winter: drag out our warm clothes, put on storm windows, and have our cars winterized for the long season ahead.

Mother continued to slip away. The only thing that remained consistent was her enormous appetite. It remained amusing to see her eat with such abandon.

"Michele, do you know when Hels will be ready to 'check out?"

"When, Mom?"

"When she stops eating."

I had come to believe that was the way it would happen.

In late summer of 1996, I made a decision to move to a new residence. I was also moving forward with my life after ending a difficult relationship.

The morning after my move in late September I visited Mother. Breakfast was being served. After the stress of the preceding weeks of work and planning the move, it was a comfort just to be in her presence. I remember saying to her, "Mom, I've moved. I am safe. Everything is all right." I am not sure she understood what I was saying, but she smiled when I touched her arm.

Two weeks passed. One evening a nurse stopped me in the hall after I had arrived to feed Mother her dinner. She said without concern, "Hels hasn't been eating the past day or so."

"Is she not feeling well?"

"Her vitals appear to be normal."

At first I thought nothing of my conversation with Michele. But as the days passed I kept hearing, "You know Chrissy, Hels isn't eating."

I started to realize that she was taking only a couple of mouthfuls at a meal for me. Then I remembered my earlier remark to Michele. Suddenly, I knew what was happening.

Mother was letting go. She had decided on some level to "check out" as I had put it months earlier. It was time for me to prepare for this final event.

It's a curious feeling. In the early days of Mother's disease I wished secretly to myself that she would stop struggling. As time went on she had stopped struggling. Now the final loss of not having her anymore was the only loss left.

She continued to show no interest in eating for the next ten days. I remember trying to feed her some oatmeal that had turned cold. She smiled a weak smile, which pleased me, and took a couple of spoonfuls. And that was it.

For the next three days she didn't even take liquids. The staff kept her mouth sponged with water, but it was only too obvious that she was dehydrating.

I got a call requesting my permission to give Mother morphine suppositories. I knew what that meant. Her body was in distress and they were doing their utmost to carry out my wishes to make her as comfortable as possible. The nurse informed me during every shift change.

As I was standing by Mother's bed in her dimly lit room one evening, a kindly young nurse came in to take her vital signs and sponge her mouth. I asked what I could expect over the next hours. Mother's breathing was becoming more labored. Her eyes were open and they followed us as we moved around her bed. I was concerned that she shouldn't suffer needlessly. I will never forget that young lady's remark as she continued caring for Mother.

"We treat our suffering animals with compassion and put them out of their misery. Isn't it a shame that we don't do the same for human beings?" I thought about the nurse's remark. She undoubtedly often attended those dying. My eyes filled with tears as I watched Mother's labored breathing. The nurse was right.

We put down our pets to end needless suffering when there is no hope for continued quality of life. But in the case of human beings, mercy killing is hotly debated. In cases reported over and over, individuals languish in vegetative states for years while relatives argue with jurisprudence to turn off the machine.

Every evening of this final week, I came to see Mother after work and then again later in the night. I sat next to her on the edge of the bed holding her hand and sang all her favorite songs. She loved "When the Saints Go Marching In" and to me it seemed like a good time for this particular song. At first I sang boldly to calm myself and then, leaning closer, softly into her ear. I hoped the sound would reach that part of her brain that understood.

Michele accompanied me to see Mother in the evenings. On Tuesday, October 22, I brought Joyce Fowler, her faithful neighbor, to say goodbye. The next day, October 23, as Mother showed signs of weakening, the staff advised us to stay near a phone. I planned to call periodically to check in.

That evening, Michele and I were eating dinner and trying to get some rest when I decided to call the desk on fourth floor. It was around nine-thirty.

"Hello, fourth floor nursing station."

"This is Chris Winter, Helen LaCaze's daughter."

"Oh yes, Chris."

"How is she doing?"

"I was down a couple of minutes ago to check her vitals. I think you should come soon."

I knew what that meant. Hastily we got into my car and sped down to Ebenezer. Nothing moved fast enough. We parked, raced up the ramp to the slow-moving double doors. Running in, we hurried to sign in at the front desk and grab the elevator.

The ward was eerily silent. Residents were in bed, and the staff were doing their nightly rounds. Calmed by the atmosphere, we walked down the hall to Mother's room. We could hear her breathing with great effort. The pool charge nurse, a gentle and sensitive Hispanic-American man came in. He listened to her vital signs and as he removed the stethoscope from his ears, he turned and said in a concerned voice, "Your mother is close." He assured us that he would be nearby when we needed him.

Moments seemed to tick by with slow deliberation. No one spoke. The room was quiet except for Mother's labored breathing. Choked with emotion, Michele held Mother's one hand and I held the other. The rest of the world seemed to disappear, as we stood by her side in the weak light over the head of the bed.

Mother's eyes were open. We stayed focused entirely on her, each taking a moment to say some last words. I bent down and hugged her saying, "I love you Mom, I will always love you. It's all right now, you can let go." I could taste the salt from my tears as I kissed her goodbye.

Michele placed her hand on Mother's chest feeling her heartbeat as she repeated over and over, "Don't go Hels, please, don't go!" She was sobbing in despair as she hugged her one last time. Mother took a few short breaths and then with one final shudder, left us.

We had the extraordinary opportunity to be with her in her final moments, truly a gift. I recognized the enormity of those last seconds. Mother had been with me at my beginning, and now I was with her at her end. She passed peacefully. As I bent down to kiss her one more time, I noticed a large tear in the corner of one eye. Whatever she experienced at that final moment, I believe, was beautiful. She had been content and ready.

It was a little after eleven o'clock. The young male nurse who had been so kind and attentive in those final hours was getting ready to go off duty. I walked over to where he stood and touched his arm.

"My mother is gone. Would you come and look in again?"

"You know, my mother told me to go to mass tonight before I came to work. She said someone would pass over and I would be needed. I was honored to serve your mother."

"You are so caring. I'm grateful you're here tonight."

Returning to Mother's room and walking over to her bed, he gently checked Mother's vital signs. When he finished he reached over and hugged me.

"Take care of each other, won't you?" He then left the room.

I told the next charge nurse what had just happened and arranged to call the Cremation Society. Upon notification of death, the organization sends someone.

Mother lay on the bed, her eyes open. I attempted to close her eyes but they wouldn't stay shut, so I let it go. After what seemed like an eternity, two aides came to the room and began preparing her.

Michele didn't want me to hold or speak to her. She needed time. Theirs had been such a special relationship. It was difficult to watch my daughter's pain at losing her grandma while I was trying to deal with my own feelings.

Michele was angry that it took so long for the Cremation Society to come for Mother. I explained to her there was only one person on duty that night and he was out making other calls when the nurse called. "Someone will be here for Hels as soon as possible, Michele."

An hour later, a gentleman arrived with a gurney to pick up Mother. He was kind, but very businesslike and gave me his card. He covered Mother and placed her on the gurney. As he wheeled her to the elevator, Michele and I followed holding hands. Michele and I gave Mother a final hug and left the building.

"Mom, can I stay the night? I don't want to be alone."

"Of course, let's go home and get some sleep,"

As we drove, the silvery light of a full harvest moon spread over the last of autumn's foliage. Just as we pulled up in front of my apartment, we heard an intriguing sound. Looking up in the star-filled night sky, we marveled at a large flock of geese flying overhead, etched in moonlight, heading south to a warmer climate. To me it was a sign that Mother had gone home.

Mother was no longer encumbered by her frail body and her diseased mind. She was once again the extraordinary spirit she had been her whole life. Boundless, independent and by her very nature, an original, Mother was now completely free.

I took comfort in all the wonderful images of her that seemed to rush through my thoughts in the days following her death. She was truly liberated, and somewhere she was dancing to a jazz beat, celebrating life in a whole new place. Helen LaCaze was truly "on the sunny side of the street."

In Retrospect 28

L ooking back over the course of Mother's illness, several thoughts come to mind. The one image that impacts me the most was her transformation from a engaging, intelligent and vital woman to a helpless, frail, silent and vacant human being caught in the vise of a debilitating disease through no fault of her own.

The mundane steps to close out the business parts of one's life seem endless. Following my mother's death, I began the long process of notifying all the involved parties. First, I called family and close friends. I got copies of the death certificate to legally notify businesses of her passing.

Next I made the necessary and pedestrian calls to the county, the Social Security Administration, the former employer who dictated her pension allotment, and the insurance company handling her monthly annuity. I had to notify them in writing as well. I closed the conservator bank account once the last check had cleared. The bank informed me, and I contacted my attorney, Mark Douglass. He informed the Court.

The memorial service was pre-choreographed. I had arranged it two years earlier when hospice workers had been called in. I had lined up the music and nine eulogizers from different stages of her life.

I reserved the chapel at the Cremation Society and ordered flowers on behalf of my cousins, Uncle Paul's offspring. I hired a trumpet soloist on Jimmy Martin's recommendation. Jimmy prepared a delightful medley of Mother's favorite songs. He would play "I Believe In You," "I'm A Brass Band," "Hi Lili, Hi

Lo," "I'll Be Seeing You," and "The Way You Look Tonight." David Englestad, the chaplain from Ebenezer, would preside at the service. After reading some of Mother's writing, he insisted on basing his sermon on her work.

It was truly a celebration of Mother's life. The room was full to overflowing with people from every part of her life's journey: from her early working days; the Order of Eastern Star; my theatre cronies; and staff from Nemer, Fieger & Associates.

Michael Tracy, a good friend, eulogized her as he read Henry Van Dyke's poem *A Parable Of Immortality*. These few words reminded me of all the good friends who had come from near and far to pay her tribute.

"And just at the moment when someone at my side says,

"There she goes!" There are other eyes watching for her coming

And, other voices ready to take up the glad shout, "Here she comes!"

These words and others gave glorious tribute to the woman who had touched so many lives, a grand farewell from all involved. Through out the service, I imagined how pleased Mother would be with all the glowing thoughts and memories shared. And of course, I thought of the symbolism in the title of the song that was her favorite, where she chose to live—on the sunny side of the street.

I waited a year to the anniversary of her passing to spread her ashes. In the interim, I developed a relationship with Paul Fournier who became my future husband. Paul had never met Mother, but from descriptions of all who had known and loved her, he said he had a clear picture of her in his mind. When I mentioned my plan to scatter her ashes on the first anniversary of her passing, Paul asked if he could accompany me to the spot I had previously picked out.

On a beautiful October morning, Paul and I walked to a small footbridge over Minnehaha Creek in Minneapolis. The early morning sky was a clear deep azure. Against this background of golden trees with the rushing creek below, I scattered Mother's ashes while Paul dropped red, yellow and orange carnations into the water.

The location was perfect. Mother loved the water and the creek would carry her remains to the Mississippi River and the river would carry her to New Orleans and the Gulf of Mexico, and even perhaps somehow to Hawaii. These were the places that had meant so much to her.

I gave a portion of Mother's ashes to Michele. She didn't wish to accompany me that day. She wanted to choose her own time and place. In the end, she chose to keep the ashes with her. I respected her decision.

Every year marking the anniversary of Mother's passing, I return to the spot on the creek in Minneapolis. I scatter flowers in her favorite colors—red, yellow and orange. For me, it is a way to remember her and celebrate her life. It reminds me that her spirit is alive somewhere in the Universe. It is a tribute to her immense persona, her gift for life and the gift she was.

On the sunny side of the street was where Mother chose to be during her journey in this life and in spite of the shade she was forced to exist in during her struggle with Alzheimer's, she remained a true spirit of joy and love. These memories are what I keep with me always. I believe Mother has achieved immortality. She's alive not only in my heart but also in the hearts of all those who knew her.

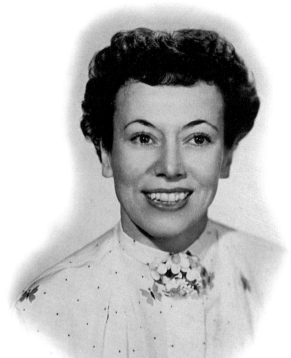

Helen Winter LaCaze
1918-1996

To My Mother

I think God must be happy
When'er he looks at you
And contemplates how faithfully
You've carried your job through
For of all of this world's mothers
There was never one so fine
So loving and devoted
As the one that I call mine

Progressive Stages of Alzheimer's Disease

This information is through the courtesy of the Alzheimer's Association Minnesota/Dakotas Chapter. Call 800-232-0851 or log on to www.alzmndak.org

(Remember as you read these stages that some symptoms will overlap, some will vary in sequence and all are likely to vary in the rate at which they progress. Some may not occur at all. The onset is subtle. Often the family is unsure anything is wrong. There will, however, generally be a continuous and progressive decline, rendering the person totally dependent on others for even the simplest daily living activities.)

STAGE ONE
COGNITIVE CHANGES
Begins with short-term memory loss

- Unable to find the right words
- Forgets familiar names and telephone numbers
- Begins to write reminders but loses notes
- Shows preference for familiar things
  (wears the same clothes and avoids going out)
- Judgment may be impaired early
  (dressing inappropriately for the weather)

PERSONALITY CHANGES
- Less sparkle, spontaneity and ambition
- Appears passive or easily angered and restless
- Indifferent to the ceremonies and courtesies of social life
- Decreased interest in environment and present affairs
- Family may be hurt because person "doesn't seem to care"

FUNCTIONAL CHANGES
- Appears vague, uncertain and hesitant in initiating action
- Can function without direction only in familiar surroundings
- Forgetfulness is disruptive to former daily routines
  (At this stage, the person is adept at covering up losses by using family members to fill memory gaps and/or blaming problems on fatigue, stress, grief, overwork and other people.)

STAGE TWO
COGNITIVE CHANGES
Greater difficulty with
- Memory
- Retention of new information
- Recall, calculations
- Decision-making and planning
- Following a story line
- Forgetful (may not pay bills, take medications, turn off the stove)
- Increased loss of learned behaviors
- Can only talk about familiar topics

PERSONALITY CHANGES
- Increased self-absorption
- Socially withdrawn
- Lack of interest in others

FUNCTIONAL CHANGES

- Deterioration of ability to initiate and sequence purposeful activities (bathing and driving)
- Sleep disturbance with restlessness at night
- Begins to neglect health and hygiene
- Needs directions to function in familiar surroundings
- Can respond to clear instructions

STAGE THREE
COGNITIVE CHANGES

- Judgment is seriously impaired
- Fails to understand the consequences of eating spoiled food, the danger of a smoke-filled room and dressing inappropriately for the weather
- Becomes disoriented to time and place
- Learned behavior deteriorates
- Invents words and is often unable to express self in speech or writing
- Asks questions over and over
- Confusion is prevalent
- The understanding of other's words is lost

PERSONALITY CHANGES

- Marked deterioration of warmth
- Following conditions may or may not surface (lethargy or hyperactivity, paranoia, aggression and hostility, delusions, sexual exposure)

FUNCTIONAL CHANGES

- The "large picture" or global loss occurs
- May need to be told each step of a former routine act (brushing teeth, getting dressed)
- May lose daily skills (buttoning a shirt, using a knife and fork)

- May walk with a shuffling gait or become glued to floor from inability to motor-plan)
- Often needs physical assistance with most activities of daily living (dressing, bathing, meal preparation)
- Needs protection and supervision

STAGE FOUR

COGNITIVE CHANGES

- Unable to speak or understand language, write or read, recognize anyone including self in the mirror
- Repeats words or actions

PERSONALITY CHANGES

- Total deterioration with the following possible symptoms: confusion, delusions, hallucinations, aggression, violent episodes, complete withdrawal or apathy

FUNCTIONAL CHANGES

Generally progresses to include

- Inability to feed self, chew or swallow
- Morbid hunger, eating everything in sight while still losing weight
- Putting everything in mouth
- Compulsively touches everything
- Seizures
- Constant chewing movements and smacking lips
- Difficulty walking, eventually becomes bedridden
- Incontinence of bowel and bladder
- Responsiveness to tactile stimuli only
- Eventually lack of response to pain stimuli and loss of consciousness
- Inability to survive without total care

DURATION OF THE DISEASE
DEPENDS ON

- Age of onset
- Individual health status
- Support systems
- Concurrent health problems
- The disease may last from a few to 20 years

Bibliography

Writing Down The Bones—Freeing the Writer Within
Natalie Goldberg
Shambhala Publishers
1986

The 36 Hour Day
Nancy L. Mace, MA
Peter V. Rabins, MD
John Hopkins University Press
1981, 1991, 1999 (Third Edition)

Winnie the Pooh
A.A. Milne
Methuen & Company, Ltd.
1926, 1973, 1998
Reprint by Mammoth; 1991

House at Pooh Corner
A.A. Milne
Methuen & Company Ltd.
1928, 1974, 1998
Reprint by Mammoth; 1991

Tales of Uncle Remus: The Adventures of Brer Rabbit
Julius Lester